Cancer Care in the Hospital

Edited by
Barry Hancock MD FRCP FRCR

YCRC Department of Clinical Oncology
Weston Park Hospital NHS Trust
Sheffield

With a Foreword by
Peter Selby

Professor of Cancer Medicine and
Director of the Imperial Cancer Research Fund
Cancer Medicine Research Unit
St James's University Hospital
Leeds

Radcliffe Medical Press
Oxford and New York

© 1996 Barry Hancock

Radcliffe Medical Press Ltd
18 Marcham Road, Abingdon, Oxon OX14 1AA, UK

Radcliffe Medical Press, Inc.
141 Fifth Avenue, New York, NY 10010, USA

British Library Cataloguing in Publication Data

A catalogue record for this book is available from the British Library.

ISBN 1 85775 120 5

Library of Congress Cataloging-in-Publication Data

Cancer care in the hospital / edited by Barry W. Hancock.
      p.   cm.
   ISBN 1-85775-120-5
   1. Cancer—Treatment.   2. Cancer—Patients—Hospital care.
 I. Hancock, Barry W.
   [DNLM: 1. Neoplasms—therapy.   2. Oncology Service, Hospital—organization &
   administration.   QZ 266 C2142 1995]
   RC270.8.C346   1995
   616.99'406—dc20
   DNLM/DLC
   for Library of Congress

Typeset by Advance Typesetting Ltd, Oxfordshire
Printed and bound in Great Britain by Redwood Books, Trowbridge, Wiltshire

23-25, 180-186, 188-196

Contents

List of contributors

Mr B D Aird, Principal Consultant
KPMG Management Consulting
1 The Embankment
Neville Street
Leeds LS1 4DW
(Formerly Chief Executive,
Weston Park Hospital NHS Trust)

Dr J D Bradshaw, Emeritus Consultant
Weston Park Hospital NHS Trust
Whitham Road
Sheffield S10 2SJ

Dr R E Coleman, Senior Lecturer in Medical Oncology
YCRC Department of Clinical Oncology
Weston Park Hospital NHS Trust
Whitham Road
Sheffield S10 2SJ

Professor A Faulkner, Professor of Communication Studies
Trent Palliative Care Centre
Sykes House
Little Common Lane
Sheffield S11 9NE

Dr M H Goyns, Senior Lecturer
Institute for Cancer Studies
Medical School
Floor G
Beech Hill Road
Sheffield S10 2RX

Professor B W Hancock, Professor of Clinical Oncology
YCRC Department of Clinical Oncology
Weston Park Hospital NHS Trust
Whitham Road
Sheffield S10 2SJ

Dr P C Lorigan, Lecturer in Medical Oncology
YCRC Department of Clinical Oncology
Weston Park Hospital NHS Trust
Whitham Road
Sheffield S10 2SJ

Dr R Nakielny, Consultant Radiologist
Central Sheffield University Hospitals
Royal Hallamshire Hospital
Glossop Road
Sheffield S10 2JF

Dr J M O'Neill, Senior Registrar in Palliative Care
Weston Park Hospital NHS Trust
Whitham Road
Sheffield S10 2SJ

Ms H C Orchard, Business Development Manager
Weston Park Hospital NHS Trust
Whitham Road
Sheffield S10 2SJ

Dr S Ramakrishnan, Consultant Clinical Oncologist
Weston Park Hospital NHS Trust
Whitham Road
Sheffield S10 2SJ

Dr R C Rees, Reader in Tumour Biology
Institute for Cancer Studies
Medical School
Floor G
Beech Hill Road
Sheffield S10 2RX

Dr M H Robinson, Senior Lecturer in Clinical Oncology
YCRC Department of Clinical Oncology
Weston Park Hospital NHS Trust
Whitham Road
Sheffield S10 2SJ

Miss C Segasby, Medical Physics Department
Central Sheffield University Hospitals
Royal Hallamshire Hospital
Glossop Road
Sheffield S10 2JF

Foreword

Hospital-based cancer care remains one of the most challenging areas of modern medical practice. Patients present to hospital doctors with a wide range of clinical features reflecting different stages of more than 100 different diseases. They will be treated by interventions which include complex and potentially hazardous surgery, high technology treatment with ionizing irradiation and/or the use of complicated, potentially toxic, drug regimens of uncertain efficacy. The teams of health care professionals responsible for looking after these patients must be able to mobilize all of the technologies for diagnosis and treatment at the same time as preserving humane and sympathetic communication with their patients throughout the patient's journey.

The team in Sheffield is deservedly well known for the breadth of its interest. Not only is there expertise in basic sciences and in complex high technology oncology but there has also been a traditional emphasis on attention to detail in the management of patients and of services and a recognition of the importance of palliative care and communication. They have brought together this expertise to produce an excellent, comprehensive text of moderate length, covering the background and management of cancer. Introductory paragraphs set the scene in epidemiology and prevention, staging and investigation. Chapters of manageable length review in general the availability of non-surgical treatments and then a systematic series of chapters cover all of the important cancer sites in up-to-date, accurate and very readable text. The final chapters cover issues of communication and palliation, emergency medicine and the management of an effective hospital-based service which will be very valuable to health care professionals and managers alike.

This is a very welcome additional text on cancer care. Its broad base, manageable length and consistency make it a very useful addition to the oncology literature.

Peter Selby
October 1995

List of abbreviations

ABMT	autologous bone marrow transplantation
ACTH	adrenocorticotrophic hormone
AFP	alpha fetoprotein
AIDS	acquired immunodeficiency syndrome
ALL	acute lymphoblastic leukaemia
AML	acute myeloid leukaemia
BCG	bacille Calmette-Guerin
BEP	bleomycin, etoposide and cisplatin
CLL	chronic lymphocytic leukaemia
CML	chronic myeloid leukaemia
CNS	central nervous system
CSF	cerebrospinal fluid
CT	computerized tomography
CTL	cytotoxic T lymphocyte
DHA	District Health Authority
DIC	disseminated intravascular coagulation
DNA	deoxyribonucleic acid
DTPA	diethylenetriamine pentaacetic acid
EAGC	Expert Advisory Group on Cancer
EBV	Epstein–Barr virus
ECG	electrocardiogram
EDTA	ethylenediaminetetra-acetate
EEG	electroencephalography
ESR	erythrocyte sedimentation rate
GFR	glomerular filtration rate
GnRH	gonadotrophin releasing hormone
GP	general practitioner
GVHD	graft *versus* host disease
HCG	human chorionic gonadotrophin
HIV	human immunodeficiency virus
HLA	human leucocyte antigen

HPOA	hypertrophic pulmonary oesteoarthropathy
HPV	human papillomavirus
HTLV	human T lymphocyte virus
IFN	interferon
Ig	immunoglobulin
IL	interleukin
IVP	intravenous pyelography
LAK	lymphokine activated killer
LVEF	left ventricular ejection fraction
MDP	methylene disphosphate
MHC	major histocompatibility
MIBG	meta-iodobenzylguanidine
MRI	magnetic resonance imaging
MUGA	multiple gated acquisition
NHS	National Health Service
NK	natural killer
NSAIDs	non-steroidal anti-inflammatory drugs
PA	posteroanterior
PBSC	peripheral blood stem cells
PLAP	placental alkaline phosphatase
PSA	prostate specific antigen
PTHRP	parathyroid hormone-related peptide
PUVA	psoralen and ultraviolet light A
PVC	polyvinyl chloride
RNA	ribonucleic acid
SIADH	syndrome of inappropriate antidiuretic hormone
SVC	superior vena cava
TGF	transforming growth factor
TNF	tumour necrosis factor
TNM	(tumour, node, metastasis) system of classification
TSH	thyroid stimulating hormone
TURP	transurethral resection of the prostate
WHO	World Health Organization

Incidence and epidemiology

M H GOYNS, B W HANCOCK and R C REES

Incidence

Impressions can be very misleading and this is especially true with respect to the incidence of malignant disease. A worker in general practice might well regard the overall incidence of cancer as low; one in a general hospital is likely to regard it as higher; one in a specialist oncology hospital might get the impression that it is very common.

In fact, in the UK about three new cases of cancer are diagnosed each year for every 1000 of the population. One in every five persons born is likely to develop some form of the disease at some time during their life. The average general practitioner (GP) will see seven new cases each year, but will see some types of malignancy very rarely. Cancer is not the most common cause of death; the annual death rate from cardiac diseases is approximately three times that from malignant disease.

Cancer registration

With the development of cancer registration schemes, accurate estimations of the incidence of the disease in general and of its different types have become possible. It has become evident that overall the incidence has changed little over the past 50 years.

The registration of new cases on presentation provides a much more accurate estimation of incidence than do mortality statistics. Successfully treated malignant disease may not contribute to an individual's death, and therefore may not feature as the certified cause of death.

Changing incidence of disease

Since the beginning of the twentieth century, there has been a steady reduction in infant mortality, due in large part to improved neonatal care, and more recently to the availability of antibiotics. Whereas the principal causes of death in early life were infectious diseases, tuberculosis and other lung diseases, malignant disease now shows a relatively increased incidence in childhood.

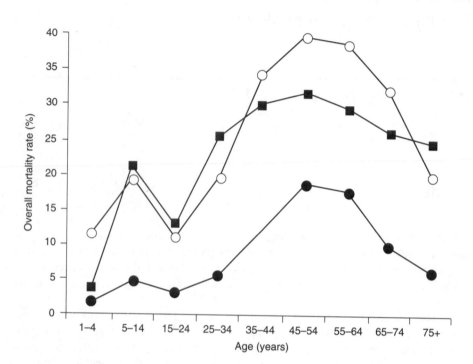

Figure 1.1 Overall mortality from malignant disease in England and Wales in 1923 (●), 1973 (■) and 1989 (○). (Based on Government Statistical Service data from *Mortality Statistics – Cause.*)

Age and sex factors

The incidence of malignancy increases with age, for most types of the disease. However, it is higher in the first 5 years of life than in the next two 5-year periods, principally due to leukaemia, to tumours of the central nervous system (CNS) and to embryonal tumours. In an increasing and ageing population, the number of patients developing the disease will increase, even though the incidence at any age remains the same and despite the fact that the chance of dying of the disease at any age is gradually decreasing. The overall incidence is the same in men and women, but the relative rates vary with age. Below the age of 10 years, it is higher in boys than in girls. In adults, 20–60 years of age, it is somewhat higher in women, especially between 35 and 50 years of age, due to the relatively high incidence of malignancy of the breast and uterine cervix. Over the age of 60 years, the incidence in men is markedly higher than that in women. Figure 1.1 reflects the overall mortality of the disease by age. For Western countries, the order of overall incidence of malignant disease for each sex and site is shown in Table 1.1 and Figure 1.2. The predominating type of malignancy also varies with age. In children of both sexes up to the age of 10 years, brain tumours and the leukaemias are most common. In men,

Men		Women	
Site	(%)	Site	(%)
Lung	25	Breast	22
Others	22	Others	26
Skin	12	Skin	11
Prostate	9	Lung	10
Bladder	7	Colon	8
Stomach	6	Ovary	4
Colon	6	Stomach	4
Rectum	5	Rectum	4
Pancreas	3	Cervix	4
Oesophagus	2	Uterus	3
Kidney	2	Pancreas	3

Table 1.1   Cancer incidence by site

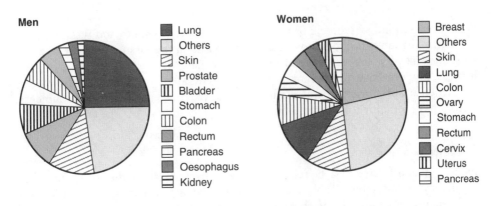

Figure 1.2   Incidence of malignant disease by site. (Based on Trent Regional Health Authority data from *Radiotherapy Statistical Tables for 1977*.)

testicular tumours are most common between 20 and 30 years, carcinoma of the bronchus from 45 to 65 years and adenocarcinoma of the prostate over the age of 70 years. In women, carcinomas of the breast and uterine cervix are most common between 25 and 65 years of age; the predominance of carcinoma of the breast persists at all ages thereafter.

Geographical factors

The incidence of malignant disease varies between different countries and different races. An outstanding example is the very low incidence of carcinoma of the uterine cervix in Jewish women. Other examples include: the very high incidence of carcinoma of the postnasal space in the Chinese; the high incidence of malignancy

Site of cancer	Professional and others		Inter-mediate		Skilled Non-manual		Skilled Manual		Partly skilled		Unskilled	
	M	F	M	F	M	F	M	F	M	F	M	F
Trachea, bronchus and lung	53	73	68	82	84	89	118	118	123	125	143	134
Uterine cervix	–	<20	–	66	–	69	–	120	–	140	–	161
Breast	–	117	–	121	–	110	–	109	–	103	–	92
Prostate	91	–	89	–	99	–	115	–	106	–	115	–

Measured in standardized mortality ratios (SMRs). The median is 100.

Table 1.2   Standardized mortality ratios by occupation in England and Wales from 1970 to 1972 (Based on Government Statistical Service data from *Social Trends.*)

of the uterus in Indian women; primary liver malignancy in South and West Africans; bladder malignancy in Egyptians; stomach tumours in the Japanese and Scandinavians; and the very low incidence of breast malignancy in the Japanese. It is of great interest, however, that immigrant populations generally tend to assume the pattern of incidence appropriate to their adopted country, suggesting that environmental factors have a major role in aetiology.

Social factors

Environmental factors may be related to local geographical conditions, or to different life styles and habits (Table 1.2). In women, the age of marriage, the number of pregnancies and the attitude to breast feeding may be relevant. To some extent, these factors may be determined by the degree of economic development of the country, and the associated social and economic status of the population, as is nicely illustrated in old data on occupational status (Table 1.2). It is becoming increasingly evident that environmental factors are responsible for many forms of malignant disease.

Industrial factors

As will be seen in more detail later, the increased risk of workers in some industries developing malignant disease is well recognized. As long ago as 1775, Percival Pott noted an association between carcinoma of the scrotal skin and chimney sweeping as an occupation. Earlier in the twentieth century, the tendency of mule-spinners to develop similar tumours became evident. This was related to the use of certain mineral oils to lubricate the spindles of the mules. More recently, an increased incidence of bladder carcinomas in workers in the azo dye industry and in the rubber and cable industries has been recognized. Workers who have prolonged contact with tar and pitch show a tendency to develop warty lesions in the exposed skin and these can progress to carcinomas. Prolonged contact with arsenical compounds can have similar effects.

Inhalation of dust containing chromates or dichromates can lead to lung malignancy. Even more active is asbestos dust, which can result in tumours of the pleura (mesotheliomas) as well as of the bronchial mucosa. Long-term inhalation of benzol vapour can result in bone marrow changes ranging from anaemia and pancytopenia to leukaemia.

Prolonged exposure of the skin to strong sunlight results in a higher than average incidence of keratotic lesions that have a marked tendency to undergo malignant change. This is seen, for example, in Indian tea planters and in Australian sheep farmers. The incidence of malignant melanoma of the skin increases with increasing exposure to natural or artificial ultraviolet light. Long periods of exposure to ionizing radiation can also induce skin malignancies. This was seen particularly in early radiation workers, some of whom accumulated relatively large doses to the hands before the dangers of radiation were recognized.

All these forms of malignant disease are related to identifiable chemical carcinogens or to physical agents that can have carcinogenic effects. Once recognized, steps can be taken to limit or prevent exposure, or to introduce alternative non-carcinogenic agents in industry.

Mortality from malignancy

For many forms of the disease, mortality rates are showing a gradual fall. This is true particularly for malignancy of the stomach, uterus, bones and tongue. Malignancy of the pharynx is showing a reduction in women but not in men. Mortality is rising for malignancy of the ovary, pancreas, bladder, kidney and lung, and for the leukaemias and the lymphomas. The increasing mortality from carcinoma of the lung (bronchus) is most striking.

The overall mortality for men is higher than that for women. This is due to the higher incidence of malignancies of lower curability in men, especially bronchial and gastric carcinomas.

Changing mortality patterns therefore reflect changes in incidence and detection and the effects of therapy on different tumours.

Aetiology

It is now generally accepted that malignant disease is genetically based. Firstly, almost all neoplasias appear to be monoclonal, that is to say, all of the malignant cells that comprise a particular tumour or leukaemia appear to have arisen from a single ancestral cell. This can be inferred from the presence of markers, such as abnormal chromosomes or enzyme isotypes. This implies that the instructions of malignancy are hereditary, as they have been passed down the generations of cells. Secondly, chromosomal changes are one of the most characteristic features of neoplastic cells and in some cases particular chromosomal abnormalities are associated with particular types of malignant disease. Thirdly, a number of tumours involve a clear inherited predisposition to neoplasia. All of these observations indicate that genes within normal cells may be altered as a prerequisite for the evolution of malignant disease.

One of the most important facts to be realized, during the past 10 years, is that environmental causes of cancer appear to act by producing genetic damage. It has been known for some time that carcinogens, be they chemical carcinogens or radiation, are mutagenic. Furthermore, the mutagenic efficiency of such agents is closely linked to their efficiency as carcinogens. What is particularly interesting is that in recent years the genetic damage caused by a range of carcinogens has been defined in great detail. It is particularly noteworthy that the genes that have been identified as being the targets of carcinogens are also the same genes that have been implicated from the studies of chromosomal abnormalities and familial malignancies. These genes are generally regarded as belonging to two groups. Those that act in a dominant fashion, in which alterations to only one allele can contribute to the evolution of a malignant phenotype, are known as oncogenes. Those that involve genes which require alterations (or deletions) of both alleles to allow for the evolution of a malignant phenotype are known as tumour-suppressor genes.

Genetic factors

Familial predisposition

Approximately 50 types of rare cancer are known to be associated with a dominant heritable predisposition. In these cases, penetrance appears to be high but the associated gene by itself is insufficient to produce a malignant phenotype, and at least one other somatic event is necessary to allow for the evolution of these particular types of cancer. An example of this situation is retinoblastoma in which two events appear to be necessary for both hereditary and sporadic forms of the disease. These events are now known to be the loss (caused by deletion or mutation) of the two alleles of the *RB1* tumour-suppressor gene that is located on chromosome 13. Several types of tumour that exhibit an inherited predisposition are summarized in Table 1.3.

Tumour	Chromosome localization of associated gene
Retinoblastoma	13q14
Multiple endocrine neoplasia (Type 1)	11q13
Multiple endocrine neoplasia (Type 2)	10q
Neurofibromatosis (Type 1)	17
Wilms' tumour	11p13
von Hippel–Lindau syndrome	3p
Nonpolyposis colorectal cancer	2p16
Polyposis colorectal cancer	5q

Table 1.3 Hereditary tumours and chromosomal localization of their associated genes

Chromosomal abnormality syndromes

In certain types of chromosomal disorders the incidence of neoplasia is increased. In Down's syndrome (trisomy 21) acute leukaemia is a well-known complication. An increased incidence of breast cancer has been observed in Klinefelter's syndrome (XXY).

Hormonal

Perhaps the most striking example of hormonal influence in cancer is in breast carcinoma. Some breast tumours are hormone responsive and this seems to correlate with the presence or absence of steroid receptor proteins in breast tissue cells. This has considerable therapeutic implications as we shall see later. It is likely that imbalance of endogenous hormones, rather than any direct oncogenic effects of these hormones, predisposes to cancer. Other examples of hormone-dependent tumours are prostatic carcinoma and carcinoma of the body of the uterus.

Environmental factors

Occupational chemical carcinogens

The most important occupational carcinogens are asbestos, arsenic, benzene, chromium, nickel and petroleum fractions (Table 1.4). It is important to remember that exposure to several of these chemicals can occur in one person's working lifetime with possible carcinogenesis of a number of tumours (e.g. lung carcinoma, mesothelioma, head and neck cancers). Historically, the soot-induced scrotal carcinoma of chimney sweeps and the aniline-dye-induced bladder cancers achieved notoriety. More recently the effects of asbestos, particularly on the lung, of industrial mineral oils on the skin and of polyvinyl chloride (PVC) on the liver have provided the main debating points on chemical carcinogenesis.

Environmental chemical carcinogens

The importance of urban atmospheric pollution (e.g. with aromatic hydrocarbons and asbestos particles) in carcinogenesis is still uncertain. The roles of arsenic in the drinking water of certain populations as a cause of skin cancer, and of aflatoxins from *Aspergillus flavus* in the staple foodstuffs of certain tropical peasants as a cause of liver cancer seem undeniable (Table 1.4). In fact, aflatoxin has now been demonstrated to be responsible for mutations in the *P53* tumour-suppressor gene in liver cancer cells. There is also a causative association between pentose-rich fibres and lower gastrointestinal malignancy, and between poor nutrition and upper gastrointestinal cancer. In fact, differences in diet probably account for more variation in the incidence of cancer than any other factor.

There are undoubtedly substances (e.g. nitrosamines) used as preservatives or colouring reagents in everyday foods, which if present in large enough quantities could be carcinogenic. The amounts present in food, however, are minute and the hazards which they present are uncertain.

Carcinogen	Type of cancer
Occupational exposure	
Asbestos	Lung
Arsenic	Skin, lung
Chromium	Lung
Nickel	Lung, paranasal sinuses
Polyvinyl chloride (PVC)	Liver
Organic chemicals	Lung, skin, bladder
Petroleum fractions	
Aromatic amines	
Benzene	
Environmental and food	
Aromatic hydrocarbons (e.g. atmospheric)	Lung
Asbestos (e.g. atmospheric)	Lung
Arsenic (e.g. in drinking water)	Skin
Aflatoxin (e.g. moulds)	Liver
Preservatives (e.g. nitrosamines)	Colon
Social customs	
Tobacco smoking	Lung, oesophagus
Iatrogenic	
Arsenic	Skin
Cytotoxic drugs	Various
Immunosuppressive drugs	Various
Exogenous hormones	Various

Table 1.4   Chemical carcinogens and cancer

Chemical carcinogens used in social customs

The main offender in this category is cigarette smoking; the carcinogenic effects of which are well known (Table 1.4). The chewing of quids (e.g. betel nuts, tobacco and burnt lime) is an important cause of oral cancer. Alcohol is thought to increase the incidence of mouth and throat cancer, particularly in smokers. It is estimated that tobacco has an aetiological role in 25–30% of all cancers. It has now been established that of the 4000 chemicals present in tobacco and tobacco smoke, 40 are known to cause deoxyribonucleic acid (DNA) mutations. It has also been established that one of the most consistent features of lung tumour cells is that they contain mutations in the K-*RAS* oncogene and the *P53* tumour-suppressor gene.

It has now been demonstrated that one of the most common genetic abnormalities in human cancer involves the *P53* gene. This gene codes for a protein which plays an important role in guarding the integrity of the genome. Therefore, when it is damaged or deleted from the cell, due to mutation, the cell becomes much more susceptible to acquiring further mutations. Interestingly, tobacco carcinogens have been found to cause mutations in a different part of the *P53* gene than aflatoxin. Therefore, *P53* gene mutations in colon cancer occur in particular regions of the *P53* gene, which are more susceptible to mutation by certain carcinogens in the diet. In lung cancers, where the incidence of such mutations of the *P53* gene accounts for only 8% of abnormalities, it has been proposed that exposure to carcinogens in tobacco smoke results in a different pattern of mutation of the *P53* gene. Until recently, it was thought that all *P53* gene mutations were functionally equivalent, but recent data have indicated that different mutations may result in distinct malignant phenotypes. This implies that the cause of lung tumours may be inferred from the type of mutation observed in the *P53* gene.

Radiation

Ionizing radiations have the capacity to displace electrons from atoms, thus converting them to ions. They can therefore cause chemical changes within living cell molecules, the most important being the damage to nuclear DNA with consequent changes in the structure and linkage of the spiral strands. If these changes are severe enough, cell death will result. Less severe changes may cause the cells to become permanently altered, in such a way as to escape normal control mechanisms (i.e. to become neoplastic).

Examples of radiation-induced tumours include: the high incidence of skin cancers in early X-ray workers; lung cancer in the miners of radioactive ores; bone tumours in girls who painted luminous watch dials with radioactive radium; thyroid cancer in people who survived atomic bomb blasts or who had neck irradiation in childhood; and leukaemia in patients with ankylosing spondylitis treated by radiotherapy. Similarly, sunlight, by virtue of its ultraviolet irradiation, may over the years cause skin cancer in fair-skinned people, by damaging DNA in the skin cells. It has now been demonstrated that these types of radiation cause mutations in genes. In particular, skin cancers containing radiation-induced mutation of the *MYC* or *RAS* oncogenes, or of the *P53* or *RB1* tumour-suppressor genes have been identified.

Viruses

A number of viruses have been implicated in animal and human cancers and leukaemias. The retroviruses (the genome of which is composed of ribonucleic acid (RNA)) have often been implicated in malignant disease in animals. However, with the exception of human T-cell leukaemia virus (HTLV-1) which is thought be a factor in the evolution of some cases of T cell leukaemia and lymphoma, these viruses do not appear to be important in human malignant disease. In humans, the viruses that have been implicated are DNA viruses, such as human papillomavirus (HPV), hepatitis B virus and Epstein–Barr virus (EBV). Viral infection by itself is often insufficient to produce a tumour. For example, 1 in 20 women infected with HPV type 16 or 18 will develop cervical cancer, 1 in 20 men infected with hepatitis B will develop liver cancer and 1 in 1000 people infected with EBV will develop lymphoma or nasopharyngeal cancer in non-endemic areas.

HPV types 16 and 18 appear to be important causative agents in cervical cancer and their tumorigenic effect is mediated by the expression of two viral proteins, E6 and E7. It has now been established that E6 interacts with the protein product of the *P53* tumour-suppressor gene and that E7 interacts with the protein product of the *RB1* tumour-suppressor gene.

The mechanism of action of hepatitis B in causing liver cancer is not so well defined, but some reports have suggested that after infection, the virus genome might integrate into the host cell genome near to one of the *ERB*-A oncogenes and alter the oncogene's expression.

EBV appears to act by immortalizing cells as a first step towards malignant transformation. The EBV-immortalized cells, however, appear to be recognized as foreign by the immune system and are usually destroyed. It is only in individuals whose immune system has been compromised in some way, for example, immunosuppressed transplant patients, patients with acquired immunodeficiency syndrome (AIDS) or possibly people who have had malaria, that these EBV-induced tumours can evolve.

Chronic irritation

Cancers can arise at sites of chronic irritation, and in relation to scars, foreign bodies and chronic inflammation. Presumably, cell damage at these sites gives rise to abnormal tissue differentiation. Oral cancer is probably the best example of this type of carcinogenesis. Factors such as pipe smoking, ill-fitting dentures, poor dental hygiene and chronic infection (e.g. syphilis) are all recognized predisposing causes for oral cancer. In carcinoma of the vagina and cervix uteri there is an aetiological association with early coitus and/or poor genital hygiene. Certain chronic diseases also predispose to human cancer. Good examples of this are achlorhydria and pernicious anaemia associated with stomach cancer; Paterson–Kelly syndrome and post-cricoid carcinoma; ulcerative colitis and colonic carcinoma; cirrhosis and hepatoma; Paget's disease and bone sarcoma; bilharzia and bladder cancer.

Iatrogenic factors

Iatrogenic (doctor-induced) chemical carcinogenesis is of uncertain importance but the effects of new medications on the population may take years to evaluate. The carcinogenic problems seen at the present time are mainly related to the use of immunosuppressive and cytotoxic drugs in cancer, transplantation and autoimmune disease, and to the use of exogenous hormones (e.g. anabolic steroids and liver cancer; prenatal oestrogens and vaginal carcinoma) (Table 1.4).

Oncogenes

The above observations have indicated that genes within normal cells may be altered as a prerequisite for the evolution of malignant disease. Such genes have become known as oncogenes. An oncogene is an altered form of a normal gene, known as a proto-oncogene. The latter are a disparate grouping of genes, some related one to another, some completely unrelated, but all capable of being altered to form an oncogene. The protein product of a proto-oncogene has an important role in normal cell physiology. It is usually involved in regulating an aspect of cell growth, apoptosis or cell differentiation.

The oncogene is abnormal in that it produces too much or too little of its protein product, or it produces an abnormal protein. By convention, each oncogene has been given a name based on a combination of three letters written in italics (e.g. MYC, RAS, SRC), although some closely related oncogenes are also distinguished from one another by an extra letter or number (e.g. MYC, MYCL, MYCN, BCL-1, BCL-2, BCL-3). Two general classes of oncogenes have been recognized. The first are the dominant-acting oncogenes (often simply called oncogenes), which require the alteration of only one of their two alleles within a cell for an oncogenic effect to occur. The second group are the recessive oncogenes (often called tumour-suppressor genes), which require that both of their alleles be deleted or mutated to allow for an oncogenic effect. There are now over 100 genes that can be classed as an oncogene or tumour-suppressor gene.

Although oncogenes are essential for the evolution of human cancer, it is important to remember that one oncogene will not cause cancer. Cancer is a multi-stage process and it is likely that an oncogene is necessary for each stage to occur. The involvement of more than one oncogene in tumorigenesis has been demonstrated by studies of colon carcinoma. It has been observed that the K-RAS oncogene occurs in a large proportion of these tumours and is usually mutated during the early stages of malignancy. Progress to full malignancy appears to depend on the mutation or deletion of the P53 tumour-suppressor gene and metastatic ability on the loss of the DCC tumour-suppressor gene. Other oncogenes are also likely to be involved in this process. Such studies are now allowing researchers to build up a framework of genetic changes that define the malignant evolution of a number of types of tumours and leukaemias.

An understanding of how the malignant cell phenotype may be defined in terms of oncogene involvement has been made possible by the discovery of the functions of the proteins coded for by the normal counterparts (proto-oncogenes) of the oncogenes and tumour suppressor genes.

As the proto-oncogenes were isolated, and as part or all of their nucleotide sequences determined, it proved possible to compare the sequences (and the amino acid sequences that they code for) with relevant computer data banks. This procedure has demonstrated that several of these protein products are identical to or have very close homology with known proteins (Table 1.5). As a result it is now possible to identify which genetic changes are necessary for the emergence of different aspects of the cancer cell phenotype.

As might be expected, uncontrolled proliferation of tumour cells is often associated with overproduction of growth factors or their receptors. It is therefore not surprising that several of the oncogenes code for such proteins. SIS codes for part of the platelet derived growth factor, ERB-B for the epidermal growth factor receptor and FMS for colony stimulating factor-1 receptor. The proliferation signal that is triggered by the action of a growth factor and its receptor is carried inside the cell by a series of proteins which eventually activate transcription factors (proteins that control the switching on or off of genes) in the cell nucleus. The RAS oncogene family have been shown to code for G-proteins that are typical of this intracellular signalling pathway and the oncogenes JUN and FOS code for subunits of the AP-1 transcription factor. In other words, all of these oncogenes (and many others beside), code for proteins that are involved in the regulation cell growth and proliferation. These observations are very important as an alteration in the structure

Oncoprotein	Function
SIS	Platelet derived growth factor
HST	Fibroblast growth factor
ERB-B	Epidermal growth factor receptor
FMS	Colony stimulating factor 1 receptor
KIT	Stem cell growth factor receptor
RAS	Membrane associated ATPase
GSP	G_s protein
SRC	Membrane-associated protein tyrosine kinase
RAF	Cytoplasmic protein-serine kinase
ERB-A	Steroid receptor
FOS	Subunit of AP-1 transcription factor
JUN	Subunit of AP-1 transcription factor
MYC	DNA binding protein
P53	DNA binding protein

Table 1.5   Function of oncogene protein products

or level of any other of these proteins could clearly contribute to uncontrolled proliferation.

The mechanism by which a cell enters apoptosis is not fully understood but a number of proteins have now been shown to be intimately involved in regulating this process. One of these proteins is coded for by the BCL-2 oncogene which can be permanently switched on in lymphocytes as a result of a chromosome trans-location. This has the effect of preventing the lymphocytes from entering apoptosis and thus increasing their cell life span, which in turn makes the lymphocytes more vulnerable to acquiring mutations in other oncogenes that regulate proliferation of these cells.

Blocks in the differentiation of cells also appear to be under the control of oncogenes. For example, in acute promyelocytic leukaemia (M3), a chromosomal translocation has been shown to alter the involvement of a glucocorticoid receptor in controlling the differentiation of these myeloid cells so that they are blocked at the promyelocyte stage of differentiation. This receptor is coded for by a member of the ERB-A oncogene family.

The induction of angiogenesis by tumour cells appears to be controlled by a number of growth factors and two that have been identified are the ligand for the ERB-B2 receptor and a member of the fibroblast growth factor family (which is coded for by the HST oncogene).

Metastasis is a complex process which is probably mediated by a range of cell adhesion molecules and growth factor signalling systems. Several proteins have now been identified that are implicated in this process. Two of these have been identified and are coded for by tumour suppressor genes. This means that both alleles of these genes are deleted or mutated and that functional protein is absent from the cell. In colon cancer it is the loss of the DCC tumour suppressor gene that is associated with metastatic spread, whereas in melanoma the loss of the NM23 gene appears to allow metastasis to occur.

Tumour biology

A tumour is formed when cells from a certain tissue escape the normal growth-regulating processes (which can involve alterations in growth control, blocks in differentiation and altered control of cell death) and proliferate more than their non-malignant neighbours. The resulting growth (neoplasm) can be either benign or malignant. In the latter case, the neoplasm has an ability to invade and destroy surrounding normal tissues and to spread to distant sites by a process known as metastasis; malignant tumours are generally termed cancers.

Tumour cells resemble normal cells in that they have the same structural features. Nuclear information is coded on the double-stranded DNA which is found in the chromosomes. The RNA is mainly concerned with protein synthesis within the cell cytoplasm. A special type of RNA (messenger RNA) conveys and translates the genetic information from the nucleus to the cytoplasmic RNA. The nucleotides are arranged in a chain-like pattern with sugar and phosphate groups, forming alternate links in the chain with nitrogenous bases (cytosine, thymine, adenine and guanine in DNA; cytosine, uracil, adenine and guanine in RNA) attached at each of the sugar units. The DNA complex is composed of two of these spiralling chains linked by hydrogen bonds across the nitrogen base units.

The unit that defines cell growth and division is called the cell cycle (Figure 1.3). The cell cycle is a continuing phenomenon in which cells that are cycling exist in a changeable equilibrium with cells that are resting (G0 phase). Cells in cycle progress either from this resting phase, or from mitosis, into a growth phase (termed G1) and then enter a period which is characterized by DNA synthesis (S phase), during which

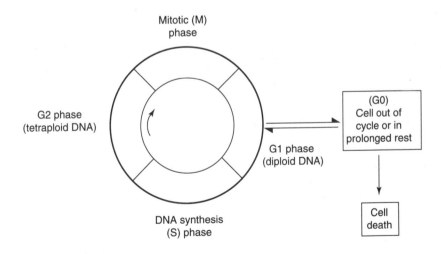

Figure 1.3 The cell cycle.

time the DNA content of the cell is doubled. The cell then progresses through a further period of growth and intracellular reorganization (G2 phase) before undergoing mitosis (M phase). During the latter, the parent cell splits into two identical daughter cells with identical DNA make-up. After this, the daughter cells may enter a further cycle or enter resting phase (G0).

Most of our information on cell cycling comes from animal cell culture experiments and such data are not always easy to translate to the *in vivo* situation. It is likely that many human cell types cycle over a period of 14–40 hours; the G1 phase is the most variable in time and thus provides the difference between fast and slowly dividing cell populations.

In the past, it was commonly accepted that tumours increased in size because they cycled more rapidly; the numerous mitotic figures seen in tumour histology sections were held to support this view. Research has now shown that tumour cell cycling times are the same as, or if anything longer than, those of normal cells. The explanation for tumour growth is in the imbalance between tumour cell formation and tumour cell loss (i.e. the failure of many tumour cells to undergo programmed cell death). New cells are added to the population at a greater rate than cells die, even though the cell loss from tumours can be considerable.

The other concept that people find difficult to understand is that usually the bigger the tumour the slower it grows (Figure 1.4). In other words, its 'doubling time', the time it takes the tumour to double its size, becomes longer because more and more cells enter G0 as the tumour grows in size. The cells left in the cycle form the tumour growth fraction, which varies from 20 to 80% in different neoplasms.

Differences in the number of cells in the resting and growth compartments and in the rate of loss of cells from the tumour account for the variations in doubling times

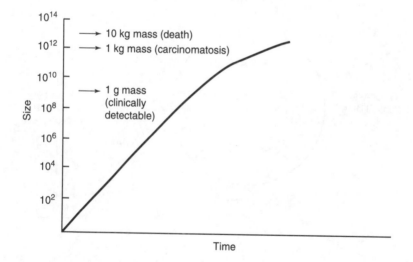

Figure 1.4 The bigger the tumour, the slower it grows.

seen in different neoplasms; leukaemias have shorter doubling times than sarcomas, and carcinomas have the longest of all.

In their development, cells need to specialize to function differently in particular tissues and organs. This process of differentiation is regulated by the genetic material coded in the DNA of the cell. Primitive cells are probably multipotent and have the potential to differentiate into many different cell types. In the tumour cell, differentiation characteristics can be lost to varying degrees. Loss of function, or gain of inappropriate function, may therefore result. The inability to recognize positional signals and the failure of contact inhibition in the tumour cells enables the cells to infiltrate normal tissues and to disseminate via blood and lymphatics to distant sites where they can survive in what should be an alien environment.

There are approximately 10^{13} cells in the human body. In its lifetime, a tumour will double its size 40 times to attain a size in excess of 1 kg, by which time there will be up to 10^{12} cells in the tumour. Unfortunately, by the time it is clinically detected a tumour will be three-quarters of the way through its growth period and there must be the equivalent of at least 1 g of tissue (10^9 cells) already present. In most patients, more than 10^{10} cells are present at the time of clinical detection. It is therefore only a further short step in the tumour's life history before 10^{12} or more cells are present and the patient dies (Figure 1.4).

Pathology

Tumours are classified according to the tissue from which they originate. They may be benign or malignant, though it must be stressed that there is considerable overlap and gradation between the two groups. The extent to which the tumour resembles its tissue of origin is noted in terms of degrees of differentiation. A tumour resembling its parent tissue will be termed well differentiated; that showing little or no resemblance will be termed poorly differentiated or undifferentiated (anaplastic). The main sites of origin and the more common types of tumour are shown in Table 1.6.

Certain histological features help to distinguish tumour tissue from normal tissue. The high mitotic activity seen in most malignant cells is more an index of the longer time spent by the cell in mitosis, with abnormal patterns of chromosomal division, than of mitotic rate, since as we have already seen, cancer cells do not divide faster than normal cells. The other histological features of malignant tumours have been noted already, including differentiation, invasion of adjacent tissues and microscopic evidence of metastases. Recognition of other more subtle microscopic changes requires the guidance of an experienced histopathologist.

Immunology

Experimental and clinical observations suggest that the immune system plays an important role in combating malignant disease. It is therefore crucial to address some of the important principles of host immunity, the discovery of human tumour antigens and the application of this knowledge in the clinical treatment of cancer.

Tissue	Neoplasm	
	Benign	Malignant
Epithelium		
Squamous	Papilloma	Squamous carcinoma
Transitional	Papilloma	Transitional carcinoma
Glandular	Adenoma	Adenocarcinoma
Connective tissue and muscles		
Fibrocyte	Fibroma	Fibrosarcoma
Fat cell	Lipoma	Liposarcoma
Muscle (smooth)	Leiomyoma	Leiomyosarcoma
Muscle (striated)	Rhabdomyoma	Rhabdomyosarcoma
Bone	Osteoma	Osteosarcoma
Vascular endothelium	Haemangioma	Haemangiosarcoma
Cartilage	Chondroma	Chondrosarcoma
Haemopoietic and lymphoreticular		
Erythrocyte	Polycythaemia vera	
Leucocyte		Leukaemia
Lymphoreticular cells	Lymphoma	Lymphoma
Plasma cell		Myeloma
Neural		
Neurocytes	Ganglioneuroma	Neuroblastoma
Glial cells	Glioma	Glioma
Nerves	Neurilemmoma	Malignant neurilemmoma
	Neurofibroma	Neurofibrosarcoma
Meninges	Meningioma	Meningiosarcoma
Embryonal and germinal		
Gonads		Seminoma
	Teratoma	Teratoma
	Hydatidiform mole	Choriocarcinoma
Kidney		Nephroblastoma
Liver		Hepatoblastoma
Neural tissue		Neuroblastoma

Table 1.6 Examples of benign and malignant neoplasms arising from various tissues

The immune system

An intact and functional immune system is required to combat infections and malignant disease. Pluripotent stem cells in the bone marrow differentiate along defined pathways where cytokines govern their expansion and maturation. T lymphocytes (cytotoxic T lymphocytes; CTL) respond in an **antigen-specific** manner and mediate the destruction of their target by recognizing a specific antigen, while natural killer (NK) cells and monocytes are **antigen non-specific** and represent a first line of defence and resistance against invading microbes and tumours. Leucocytes, such as neutrophils, kill target cells and microbes by phagocytosis, while lympho-cytes (including CTL and NK cells) either induce programmed cell death (apoptosis) or release lytic enzymes (e.g. perforin and serine esterases) which lyse cells by inducing pore formation in the cell membrane. CTLs in particular are essential in combating viral disease and cancer. B lymphocytes, which differentiate into antibody-producing plasma cells, are responsible for humoral immunity, and the resulting antibody is capable of mediating target cell destruction by combining with lytic components of the complement cascade, or with neutrophils, NK cells, mono-cytes and macrophages. When associated with cells, the antibody provides the spec-ificity for antigen recognition, while the associated leucocytes provide the armament for target cell destruction.

Using monoclonal antibody staining techniques, different leucocyte subpopula-tions can be identified. This has resulted in the identification of T helper (Th) cells (CD4$^+$) and T cytotoxic cells (CD8$^+$). In addition, Th cells are subdivided into Th-1 and Th-2 populations producing molecules (cytokines), which either promote growth and differentiation of immunocytes or restrict the development of immunity, respectively. Immunodeficient states may arise through the overproduction of sup-pressor cytokines from Th-2 cells or the restricted production of Th-1 cytokines. Indeed, we have come to recognize that the interplay between cells of the immune system is mediated primarily through cell–cell contact, which triggers the release of several interactive cytokines. The development of antigen-specific immunity occurs as the result of clustering of immunocytes in lymphoid tissue, in particular between cells capable of presenting the antigen (known as antigen-presenting cells) and either T or B lymphocytes. Lymphocytes then become activated and form antigen-specific clones which populate lymphoid tissue throughout the body.

Cytokines

We now recognize more than 50 cytokines, essential for the development of antigen-specific immunity and natural resistance. They may be divided into the interleukins (IL), tumour necrosis factors, interferons, colony-stimulating factors, chemokines, growth factors and suppressive factors (Table 1.7). Cytokines may be divided simply into those which act as growth factors, such as IL-2, IL-4 and IL-12 (which induce T cell proliferation) and IL-4 and IL-5 (which contribute to B cell growth and differentiation) and those factors which restrict the development of immune

Interleukins	1–15
Interferons	αβγ
Colony-stimulating factors (CSF)	Granulocyte-CSF, macrophage-CSF granulocyte macrophage-CSF
Chemotactic cytokines (chemokines)	α β
Transforming growth factor-β	β 1–3
Growth factors (GF)	Platelet derived GF, epidermal GF FGF (fibroblast growth factor)

Table 1.7 Recognized cytokines

function and cell growth (e.g. IL-10, IL-4, transforming growth factor-β (TGF-β)). Others are involved in the proliferation and differentiation of bone marrow cells (e.g. colony-stimulating factors (CSFs)), and chemokines promote cell motility and migration. Cytokines have multiple functions, as illustrated by interferon, which is capable of inhibiting cell proliferation, enhancing NK and T lymphocyte killing, and mediates antiviral activity. IL-4 can induce T cell and B cell proliferation in response to an antigen, but is immunosuppressive towards NK cells, and can inhibit their activation by other cytokines. One cytokine prominent as a therapeutic agent in cancer is IL-2, which *in vivo* and *in vitro* has been shown to enhance antigen non-specific cytotoxicity mediated primarily by NK cells and is a principal cytokine promoting antigen-specific T cell reactivity. The involvement of IL-2 and other cytokines in cancer immunotherapy will be discussed separately in Chapter 6.

Immune surveillance

A controversial issue which remains largely unsubstantiated by direct evidence is whether or not the body maintains a continuous surveillance for the development of abnormal and potentially neoplastic cells. Theoretically, tumours consist of abnormal cell types which express new/novel antigens which may be recognized by the immune system. Antigen-specific CTL, together with NK cells and macrophages, recognize abnormal cell types, and have the capacity to destroy newly arising cancer cells. Indirect evidence substantiates this view, since patients with congenital immune deficiency disease are recognized as having an increased risk of developing cancer. Patients on immunosuppressive therapy and patients with Hodgkin's disease treated with cytotoxic chemotherapy are particularly prone to developing certain types of malignancy. It is well recognized that cancer patients have a reduced immune status, which can leave them susceptible to microbial infections; patients with advanced neoplastic disease more readily accept homograft transplants than do normal 'immunocompetent' individuals.

Tumour antigens

The enthusiasm for using immunotherapy to treat cancer has waxed and waned over the past 20 years. Observations in experimental animal models have clearly shown that tumour antigens exist which promote high levels of immunity against tumour challenge. It must be realized, however, that most of the animal tumours studied were induced with high levels of carcinogen or oncogenic viruses, and such cancers are likely to express 'new' proteins that act as potent immunogens. However, these early studies provided the impetus to develop knowledge of human tumour antigens. In certain animal models, the tumour antigens have been well characterized (for example the P815 mastocytoma and the Meth-A sarcoma systems) and tumour-specific immunity has been closely associated with the development of antigen-specific T lymphocyte reactivity or CTL. In the main, the induction of tumour-specific antibody appears to play a minor role in combating tumour growth, although antigen-non-specific immune defence mechanisms, especially NK cells, appear to mediate destruction of tumour cells in the bloodstream and reduce the incidence of tumour metastases and the development of secondary disease. CTLs are potent mediators of anti-cancer immunity and in murine models the adoptive transfer of tumour-specific CTL into mice with established tumours causes the complete regression of these cancers.

It has taken many years, and the application of recent immunological and molecular techniques, to identify antigens expressed on human cancers which potentially could act as targets for immune attack. A notable example of advancement in this field has come from the cloning of the *MAGE* (melanoma antigen) genes from human melanoma. Other antigens, capable of evoking CTL responses, are expressed on human cancer cells; these include Melan-A, gp-100 and tyrosinase. Under appropriate *in vitro* conditions, these antigens can induce CTLs which mediate the destruction of cancer cells. In addition, mutated oncogenes or tumour-suppressor genes may give rise to mutated proteins capable of acting as immunogens, which constitute potential target antigens for immune attack. That the immune system can be activated against antigens expressed on human tumours has allowed us to formulate a strategy for developing tumour vaccines for treating human malignant disease (see Chapter 6). Major histocompatibility (MHC) antigens are required for the immune system to recognize tumour antigens. The absence of MHC class I antigens results in the failure of T cells to recognize the tumour, and is a means whereby tumours escape immune destruction.

In addition to the recently discovered human tumour antigens, several other tumour-associated proteins have been discovered over the years. For example, carcinoembryonic antigen is known to be preferentially expressed in colon carcinoma as well as in other tumour types, but expressed at low levels in cells from normal individuals. Alpha fetoprotein (AFP) is also found in normal individuals, particularly during pregnancy, but elevated levels are produced during liver carcinogenesis, as well as by other tumours, particularly teratomas. These antigens do not serve as 'tumour rejection' antigens, but are of value as markers of malignant disease. In this context, human chorionic gonadotrophins (HCG) are of considerable value in monitoring trophoblastic tumours (e.g. choriocarcinoma, teratoma).

The advent of monoclonal antibodies has been of value in developing assays to identify specific proteins, especially those associated with specific cell populations. Antibodies developed against tumour-specific markers could have a role in targeting cytotoxic drugs to the tumour site, or aid in the identification of residual tumour deposits in the body. Labelling monoclonal antibodies appropriately with cytotoxic drugs or radiolabels has met with limited success, in part due to the inability of antibody molecules to penetrate tumour tissue and the limitations of conventional detection systems. Nevertheless, this approach to cancer treatment and detection is under continual review and new technologies may well develop to the point where they are clinically useful.

Immunodeficiency

Immunodeficiency is a problem in many patients with cancer, particularly those with lymphoreticular disease or disseminated disease. Immunosuppression is associated either with the cancer itself, or with the treatment given, and in many cases immunotherapy and aggressive chemotherapy induce severe immune suppression. Tumours and host cells produce immunosuppressive factors such as TGF-β, which decreases both antigen-specific and antigen-non-specific immunity. Infections are therefore not uncommon in cancer patients with widespread disease or those undergoing therapy. The organisms responsible may cause only mild symptoms in normal healthy individuals, but in contrast, cause severe and often fatal illness in immunodepressed patients. Herpes zoster, *Candida albicans*, varicella and common bacteria are the usual offenders, but more exotic infections, such as *Aspergillus*, *Cryptococcus* or *Pneumocystis*, can occur.

The decreased immunocompetence of T lymphocytes, NK cells and macrophages, together with an altered cytokine profile can lead to a state of immunological anergy in patients. Boosting the patient's immunity against infection is potentially valuable, but often difficult in those receiving continual chemotherapy or radiotherapy for their disease. It was originally believed that excessive antibody production and the presence of blocking factors produced by tumour cells contributed to the immuno-suppressive state. It is, however, more likely that cytokines such as TGF-β, IL-4 and IL-10, produced by tumour cells or host cells, mediate depressed immunity. The lack of production of those cytokines responsible for bone marrow cell development (CSFs) and cytokines involved in increasing lymphoid cell proliferation and differ-entiation (e.g. IL-2, IL-3, IL-5, IL-12), and those molecules which alter the functional capacity of lymphoid cells (e.g. interferon-gamma (IFN-γ) as a macrophage-activating factor) and IL-2, IL-12 and IFN-α/β, which increase the cytolytic activity of NK and T cells, are important aspects of immunosuppression. The role of immunotherapy in the treatment of cancer is discussed in Chapter 6.

Effects of cancer

Cancers exert their effects in three main ways: by expansion and infiltration at their site of origin; by distant spread (metastasis); and by their remote (non-metastatic, para-neoplastic) effects (Figure 1.5). Each type of neoplasm shows these effects in differ-ent degrees. Sarcomas tend to infiltrate extensively locally before metastasizing; certain differentiated thyroid tumours are notorious for metastasizing early (the follicular type via the bloodstream, the papillary type via the lymphatics); and cer-tain tumours, particularly bronchial carcinoma, can produce inappropriate hormones such as adrenocorticotrophic hormone (ACTH) as a remote effect early in their development.

The paraneoplastic (non-metastatic, remote) effects of cancers are discussed in Chapter 16. They occur in many patients (more than 15%), particularly those with widespread disease, but are sometimes not recognized. The most common offending tumour is the bronchial carcinoma, particularly the 'oat cell' type.

Cancer management

The ideal way to defeat cancer is to prevent it. As we have indicated, environmental factors are extremely important in the aetiology of tumours, thus education about these factors and avoidance of them would possibly lower the incidence.

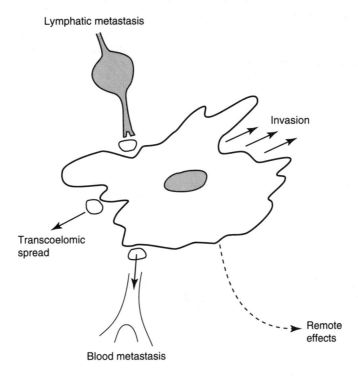

Figure 1.5   The spread of cancer.

The large number of cells (10^9–10^{10}) present when the patient is first diagnosed with cancer makes the problem of treatment difficult. Early detection by simple screening techniques, if this were feasible, would certainly help this problem. The investigation and treatment of cancer involves the GP, the hospital clinician, the radiologist and the pathologist and utilizes many other laboratory services. A full history with examination will reveal the probable diagnosis in most patients. Cancer must be confirmed, however, by biopsy and histological examination of appropriate tissues. Further investigations may be necessary to determine the extent of the disease. These include haematological, biochemical and immunological blood investigations, radiology and radioisotope scanning.

In management, the team approach is vital. The surgeon, radiotherapist and physician are all intensively involved. Any therapy must involve treating the tumour, if that is possible, and treating the patient. Attention given to communication with the patient and his or her relatives will improve morale, allay fear and inspire confidence. All these factors make for better tolerance of what may be very uncomfortable treatment.

With curable tumours, doctors can give, and patients can accept, traumatic therapy in the knowledge that a good result is possible. With an incurable lesion, such physical and mental trauma is not justified and it is far better to help the symptoms with the minimum possible disturbance to the patient's remaining daily routine – the essence of cancer palliation.

2

Education, screening, prevention and surveillance

P C LORIGAN and B W HANCOCK

Of potentially greater importance than the treatment of established cancers is the need for prevention and early diagnosis.

Education

In patients with cancer, fear is a significant cause of delay in seeking medical advice. This fear is easily understood, because many people still regard all forms of cancer as incurable. It is of great importance to stress that many forms of cancer are curable, if detected at an early stage, and that these cure rates for early cancers are being further improved by the use of extra (adjuvant) treatment at the time of diagnosis. Adjuvant treatment in common cancers can save a significant number of lives each year. Table 2.1 shows the 5-year survival rates of a number of common cancers when detected and treated at either an earlier or a later stage. In general, 5-year survival figures are a reasonable indication of long-term survival.

Apart from fear, there are a number of other reasons why patients with cancer may present with advanced rather than early disease. Ignorance, misconception and embarrassment are significant factors. People may mistakenly believe that a lump is only important if it is painful, or that an 'ulcer' is due to poor hygiene. The mass media play an increasingly important role in educating the general public about cancer, but rely in the main on fairly general and dogmatic statements. Other forms

	Early (%)	Late (%)
Invasive cervix uteri (squamous)	75–80	5
Larynx	90	20
Breast	75	5–10
Bladder	70	4–30
Colorectal	90	<30

Table 2.1   The 5-year survival rates in cancers detected early or late

of education, for example women's groups, can usefully target individuals at risk and give good quality personalized advice, but cannot hope to reach the number of people reached by the mass media. It is obvious that all these forms of education have their part to play if we wish to improve the general public's appreciation of the need to detect and act on symptoms and signs of cancer at an early stage. From a purely monetary viewpoint, education programmes are expensive, but failure to pick up cancer at an early stage results in major expenditure on the treatment of advanced disease and loss of earning capacity by the patient.

Screening

The basic principle of screening healthy people for cancer is that tumours are detected at an earlier stage, when the tumour load is lower and so easier to eradicate. This is a premise which is well founded on basic principles of cancer treatment. The major benefits of screening are that more people are cured of the disease than would be otherwise, and that this cure is achieved using less radical and less costly treatment. In addition, those who are found to be 'all clear' are reassured. There are however, many disadvantages to screening. Patients with 'borderline' abnormalities, which would normally have regressed, may be overtreated. There are problems with false-positive and false-negative test results and patients are labelled as having a disease for longer, since it is caught earlier in its natural history. In addition, the cost of screening must be taken into account.

Screening tests must satisfy a number of criteria. They must be sensitive (i.e. detect most people who have the disease) and specific (only test positive when the disease is present). Ideally the test should be validated in randomized studies. The test should be cheap and simple to carry out, be easy to interpret and should be reproducible. There must be a facility to act on positive results promptly and a well-designed course of action available for borderline results. The ideal frequency of screening must be determined and the general population must be aware of this.

The complexity of screening tests ranges from the simple cervical smear to sophisticated investigations, such as endoscopy. More complex and expensive techniques limit their general applicability to screening programmes, but are very powerful tools in small high-risk populations.

Mammography has proved useful in screening women aged 50–65 years for breast cancer and there is now a national UK screening programme for these women. It is currently being assessed in younger 'at risk' patients.

Our understanding of the molecular basis of cancer is increasing rapidly. We have already identified and cloned a number of genes implicated in many familial cancers. Over and above this we have identified a number of genes (i.e. oncogenes and tumour-suppressor genes) that are contributory factors in the development of cancer. It is fair to assume that our ability to screen for the potential for developing cancer will increase greatly over the next 10 years. The practical, moral and ethical issues that this will raise will be considerable.

Prevention

It is now well established that a number of agents are carcinogenic. Reference was made in Chapter 1 to known occupational carcinogens. The case is less clear for a number of dietary factors, atmospheric factors and pollutants. A number of viruses have been implicated in carcinogenesis; these include hepatitis B, EBV and the human immunodeficiency virus (HIV). Vaccines for a number of these have been developed. Direct physiological manipulation is being attempted in some malignancies, for example tamoxifen is given to high risk pre-menopausal women to prevent breast cancer. Gene therapy may have a role in the prevention of hereditary cancers, but this would involve germ line manipulation and many people consider this unethical. Despite all the expensive new techniques which may have a role to play, we are still finding it difficult to effect the cheapest and most effective methods, such as stopping smoking.

Surveillance

In assessing the need for follow-up surveillance in patients after treatment, three factors are important:

- knowledge of the biology of the tumour
- the advantages and disadvantages of follow-up for the patient and the doctor
- the importance of teamwork.

The behaviour of many malignancies is now understood and is predictable. They may be potentially curable (e.g. children's tumours, lymphoma and uterine carcinoma), usually incurable (e.g. lung, brain) or may have a very long natural history (e.g. breast, ovary).

In favour of follow-up is that the patient and clinician have the psychological reassurance that all is well, that the patient will be seen at an early stage of any recurrence of disease and that accurate follow-up allows accurate statistics. Against follow-up is the possibility that the patient may be anxious or uneasy about continuous follow-up, that cured patients will be followed unnecessarily, that follow-up is time consuming and that even if things do go wrong the clinician cannot always correct them.

The value of community services in follow-up cannot be overemphasized. Various community staff (e.g. GPs, nurses and social workers) play an important role, particularly when they work in close contact with the hospital oncology service.

All things considered, it is usually accepted as important for a senior hospital oncologist to supervise the follow-up of patients with close communication with other hospital specialists and with the community health team. The oncologist should know his patient well and detect slight, but significant, changes each time he sees the patient when a short history is taken and relevant examination done. Malignant disease is now accepted as the great mimic and any symptom or sign should be taken as relevant to the primary cancer or its treatment until proved otherwise. The psychological aspects of follow-up are important. Some patients will be followed unnecessarily whereas others may be well for periods from weeks to decades after therapy. Patients may not seek medical advice spontaneously but when abnormalities are found at follow-up there is a good chance that something positive can be done, possibly with further curative therapy, if not with palliative measures.

3

Staging and investigation

R NAKIELNY, C SEGASBY and B W HANCOCK

Staging cancer

It has long been known that survival is longer for local than for widespread cancer. The concept of 'staging' has been applied to many tumours and individual staging procedures will be discussed in relation to specific cancers. However, there may be different staging procedures (clinical, surgical, radiological and pathological) for the same tumour, and this makes analysis and comparison of different treatment regimens and survival figures extremely difficult. The TNM system of classification was devised in an attempt to standardize staging by using basic principles applicable to all sites regardless of therapy. It enabled further information (histopathological, surgical) to be supplemented later to the initial clinical staging. The three components of the system are T (0–4), the extent of the primary tumour, N (0–4), the condition of regional lymph nodes, and M (0–1), the absence or presence of distant metastases. Two categories of TNM classification are established, the pre-treatment clinical TNM and post-surgical histopathological p.TNM.

The TNM system has not been universally accepted, however, since the classifications for some tumours appear lengthy and sometimes cumbersome. It is nevertheless an attempt to rationalize many diverse staging procedures under one unifying concept.

Investigations

The staging of the patient depends on a full clinical and histopathological investigation. Some simple and baseline investigations are essential, and more complex procedures may also be necessary, depending on the site and type of tumour and on the age and general condition of the patient. A young, relatively fit, patient with a potentially curable lesion will require much more extensive investigation than an elderly ill patient with an incurable solid tumour. Investigations are basically of four types: tissue biopsy; blood sampling; radiology; and isotopic.

Tissue biopsy

The diagnosis of malignant disease must be established by the histological examination of a biopsy specimen from clinically involved tissue.

Blood sampling

Haematological investigations

A full peripheral blood count with examination of a blood film is mandatory in all patients with cancer. The erythrocyte sedimentation rate (ESR) is still one of the most important markers of disease activity, especially if monitored serially. Anaemia is common in malignancy. The blood film will give clues as to the nature of the anaemia, for example: the microcytic hypochromic anaemia of blood loss; the normocytic normochromic anaemia of chronic disease; the leucoerythroblastic picture of bone marrow replacement by tumour; and the macrocytic anaemia of folic acid deficiency.

The nature and differential count of peripheral white blood cells is also helpful. The presence of abnormal white cells in leukaemia or non-Hodgkin's lymphoma may suggest the diagnosis. Neutrophilia is sometimes a feature of widespread malignancy, as well as of bacterial infection. Neutropenia, lymphopenia and thrombocytopenia occur with widespread disease, either as a toxic non-specific effect or as a result of bone marrow infiltration. Thrombocytosis is another non-specific effect of malignancy. Other haematological investigations, which may be indicated, are: bone marrow examination as an aid to diagnosis of peripheral blood film abnormalities; serum ferritin to assess iron storage status; coagulation screening and platelet function studies in cases of thrombosis or bleeding; and red blood cell survival and autoantibody studies in cases of haemolysis.

Biochemical investigations

Blood samples should be taken for liver function tests (serum bilirubin, liver enzymes, alkaline phosphatase and proteins) and for urea, creatinine, calcium, uric acid and electrolyte assessment. Clinical assessment of hepatic involvement by cancer is difficult. Hepatomegaly with deranged liver biochemistry does not mean pathological involvement by tumour, and conversely hepatic infiltration may be present in the absence of hepatomegaly and when the liver biochemistry is normal. Elevated levels of serum lactate dehydrogenase indicate marked disease activity.

Immunological investigation

The importance of the immune response in cancer was discussed in Chapter 1. Assessment of immunological status in the patient with cancer is, however, optional since there is no conclusive proof that it relates to prognosis, and the various tests involved are time consuming and sometimes difficult to interpret. Assessment may be important in patients with recurrent or serious problems with infection, or in those with tumours arising from 'immune' cells (leukaemia, lymphoma and myeloma).

Radiological investigations

Chest X-ray

Radiological examinations are very important in the assessment of patients with cancer but should only be used when there are good clinical indications. It is probably necessary for most patients to have a chest X-ray because this may identify metastatic disease simply and cheaply and obviates the need for more complex investigations. It may show mediastinal/hilar lymph node involvement, pulmonary nodules or infiltration, effusions and pleural metastases. Skeletal metastases may also be visualized. A standard postero-anterior (PA) X-ray is usually the only view required. Other views such as a lateral are only taken to answer specific problems raised on the PA film.

Skeletal radiographs

The primary indication for a skeletal radiograph is bone pain. The radiographs are limited to the site of pain. Metastatic bone lesions from tumours such as breast, bronchus, prostate and myeloma are much more common than primary bone malignancies. A full skeletal survey is only required in myeloma, as all the other metastases usually show up on a radioisotope bone scan (see below).

Gastrointestinal radiographs

Barium can be swallowed to visualize the oesophagus (barium swallow), the stomach (barium meal) and the small bowel (small bowel follow through or enema). It can be injected via a rectal catheter to visualize the colon (barium enema). These, together with endoscopy techniques, can be used to investigate dyspepsia, change in bowel habit, unexplained iron-deficiency anaemia or bleeding *per rectum*. Adequate bowel preparation is vital if lesions are not to be obscured by food residue.

Ultrasound

This is a simple, cheap and, in skilled hands, a very accurate method of assessing many different body areas. It is often the first-line cross-sectional imaging method, with more expensive investigations such as computerized tomography and magnetic resonance imaging (see below) reserved for specific indications. A high frequency (3.5–10 MHz) 'real-time' probe is used to produce images in a non-invasive way. No radiation is used. Ultrasound has many uses, but in oncology the main ones are to locate and monitor abdominal masses, liver and lymph node metastases. It is very sensitive in the detection of hydronephrosis of the kidneys due to obstruction of the urinary tract. Superficial masses and testicular tumours are best assessed with high frequency ultrasound (7.5–10 MHz). Ultrasound also detects pericardial and pleural effusions and ascites. It can be used to guide biopsy of abdominal masses and drainage of fluid in the chest or abdomen.

Computerized tomography

Computerized tomography (CT) is a method of producing cross-sectional images of any part of the body using X-rays. The patient lies on a special table which moves through a gantry at selected increments (usually 1 or 2 cm) and 'slices' are taken in each position by an X-ray tube rotating around the patient. The slice thickness is controlled by the thickness of the fan-shaped 'curtain' of X-rays. It can be as little as 1 mm, but this would be very time consuming if the chest and abdomen are being investigated. In practice, the slice thickness is usually 1 cm. When the X-rays pass through the patient they are absorbed in different amounts by the various body tissues (e.g. bone absorbs a lot of X-rays whereas air in the lungs absorbs very few). The emerging X-rays are then converted into electrical signals by a bank of detectors situated on the other side of the patient opposite the X-ray tube. Computers analyse these signals and convert the data into a digital image which can then be manipulated to visualize bone, soft tissue and lung. Modern scanners have a wide (70 cm) gantry aperture so claustrophobia is seldom a problem.

Very little patient preparation is required for a CT scan. If the abdomen is being scanned the patient will usually be required to drink a litre of very dilute contrast medium 1 hour prior to the scan, so that the bowel is opacified, otherwise loops of bowel can mimic a mass. The examination takes 20–40 minutes, and the patient must be able to lie flat and not move during this time.

CT scanning is used to stage many tumours (particularly lymphoma and testicular tumours) and also to monitor the effect of treatment. It is also used to plan radiotherapy treatment, to maximize the dose to the tumour and to minimize the dose to normal tissue. It is important to remember that CT is not tissue specific. Therefore, it cannot reveal what is causing an abnormality, but it can be used to guide percutaneous needle biopsies to obtain tissue to make a definitive diagnosis. Also, microscopic tumour deposits in normal-sized lymph nodes will not be detected.

Magnetic resonance imaging

When a patient is placed in a very strong homogeneous magnetic field all the protons (weak magnets) in the hydrogen atoms of the water molecules in the body align with the applied magnetic field. A radio frequency pulse can then be applied to excite these protons and cause them to oscillate around the axis of the magnetic field like spinning tops. In effect, they act as oscillating weak magnets which induce electrical signals in receiver coils placed around the body. By tilting the applied magnetic field, protons at each point in the volume being imaged will oscillate at slightly different resonant frequencies and by 'tuning' the receiver coils through these frequencies (like tuning a radio) the strength of signal from each point in the imaged volume can be detected and hence an image produced. The physics of this imaging method is very complex. It is sufficient to know that the two major types of image produced are called T1 and T2 and depend on the way the signal decays in the longitudinal and transverse directions, respectively. T1 images have good spatial resolution (i.e. show anatomy well) but have poor contrast resolution (i.e. are not so good at detecting pathology). Conversely, T2 images have poor spatial resolution but good contrast resolution.

The patient must lie in quite a narrow tubular aperture for magnetic resonance imaging (MRI) so claustrophobia can occasionally be a problem. The switching of the gradient magnetic fields can be very noisy. A typical examination will take approximately 30–45 minutes, but can be much faster in certain circumstances.

The great advantage of MRI, apart from the fact that no radiation is used, is that images can be produced in any plane. It is also the most sensitive imaging method for detecting abnormal tissue. Unfortunately it may not be possible to say with certainty what is causing the abnormality. Its major uses in oncology are assessing spinal cord compression, brain tumour, gynaecological, bone and soft tissue malignancies. This imaging method is developing rapidly and in future other applications will be found. Patients who have a cardiac pacemaker, metallic foreign body in the eye or a cerebral aneurysm which has been surgically clipped cannot be scanned. Other metal objects in the body, due to previous surgery (e.g. clips, hip prosthesis) can usually be safely scanned 6 weeks after surgery. If in doubt, contact the MRI Department for advice.

Renal radiography

Intravenous pyelography (IVP) has now been replaced by ultrasound in most cases, because it is quicker, cheaper and less hazardous (1 in 40 000 mortality with intravenous contrast examinations). Ultrasound is particularly good at detecting hydronephrosis secondary to obstruction.

Lymphography

This technique was used to locate abdominal lymph node deposits by injecting dye into lymphatic vessels in the feet. It is time consuming, unpleasant for the patient and may be difficult to interpret. In lymphoma and testicular tumour staging it has been replaced by CT. It is occasionally used in the staging of carcinoma of the cervix.

Arteriography

The injection of contrast medium into arteries is rarely required in malignant disease.

Mammography

The radiological investigation of breasts is important in locating breast lumps and can give an indication of the likelihood of malignancy.

Interventional radiology

There are several interventional techniques that have an application in oncology. Metal stents can be used in the superior vena cava (SVC) (inserted via a venous catheter) to open it up when it is compressed by malignant tissue. Obstructed kidneys can be drained by the percutaneous insertion of a nephrostomy tube, although this has to be fully discussed if the obstruction is due to end-stage malignancy. A gastrostomy tube can be inserted through the anterior abdominal wall into the stomach to allow better feeding of patients with tumours obstructing the pharynx or oesophagus. These techniques are very specialized and can only be performed after proper consultation with the radiologists or surgeons.

Nuclear medicine investigations

In nuclear medicine, clinical information is derived from observing the distribution of a radiopharmaceutical administered to the patient. Measurements can be made of this distribution by determining the amount of radioactivity present. These measurements can be carried out either *in vivo* or *in vitro*.

In vivo imaging is the most common type of procedure in nuclear medicine, nearly all imaging being carried out by a gamma camera. Its main strength lies in the fact that it demonstrates function rather than simply anatomy.

In vitro measurements are made on samples of material taken from the patient, such as blood and urine, to determine the amount of radiopharmaceutical present. Such measurements are made using gamma or beta sample counting techniques.

Many nuclear medicine procedures provide complementary diagnostic information to other imaging modalities such as X-ray CT, ultrasound and MRI. In some cases, for example thyroid carcinoma and phaeochromocytoma, radionuclide imaging can provide a specific diagnosis. However, the relatively poor anatomical resolution of radionuclide imaging, compared with other techniques, has resulted in a decline in the clinical demand for some investigations, such as brain and liver imaging. The introduction of newer functional radiopharmaceuticals outlining tumour physiology has rejuvenated the role of nuclear medicine in clinical oncology.

Bone scanning

Bony lesions are usually associated with increased local metabolism of calcium and osteoblastic activity, demonstrable by increased uptake of a suitable tracer. Increased uptake is seen in primary or metastatic tumours, inflammation, Paget's disease and fractures. The main indication for bone scanning in oncology is for bone pain and the primary assessment of tumours that tend to metastasize early (e.g. prostate carcinoma).

The radiopharmaceutical used is a phosphate complex (e.g. methylene disphosphonate; MDP) labelled with technetium-99m (^{99m}Tc). Imaging is carried out 2–4 hours after intravenous injection and the patient is encouraged to drink plenty of fluids between injection and scan to encourage washout of any tracer not bound to the skeleton. Increased local uptake (a 'hot spot') indicates disease. Bone imaging is a more sensitive detector of local changes in the bone metabolism than X-ray or CT imaging (lesions are generally visible on X-ray after 50% of calcium is lost) but is not usually specific for particular disease processes.

Thyroid scanning

Thyroid scanning is used mainly for the elucidation of thyroid nodules and goitres and for assessment with a view to radionuclide therapy. The radiopharmaceutical commonly used is ^{99m}Tc in the pertechnetate form. It is taken up by the thyroid iodide trap, but is not incorporated into hormone. Imaging takes place 20 minutes after intravenous injection of the radiopharmaceutical.

Thyroid nodules with increased uptake are described as 'hot', they are usually autonomous and related to hyperthyroidism. 'Cold' nodules with reduced uptake indicate a cyst, neoplasm or inflammation. Further investigations are required to determine the nature of a 'cold' nodule.

Radioiodine is used when imaging with ^{99m}Tc-pertechnetate is unsatisfactory or when radioiodine ablation therapy is proposed (see Chapter 4).

Lung scanning

The most common clinical indication for lung scanning is pulmonary embolism. While it is not directly related to oncology it is as likely to occur in this group of patients as in any other and prompt diagnosis is required.

A combined ventilation/perfusion (V/Q) lung scan is required for reliable diagnosis. Gases and particulate agents are available for the ventilation scan. Gases include krypton-81m and xenon-133. Particulate agents include ^{99m}Tc-technegas and aerosol particles of ^{99m}Tc-DTPA (diethylenetriamine pentaacetic acid). While the advantage of ^{99m}Tc is that it is readily available, a possible disadvantage of particles is central deposition in patients with chronic obstructive airways disease. The patient breathes in the radiopharmaceutical and four to six views of the lung are taken. The perfusion phase is carried out after intravenous injection of ^{99m}Tc-labelled macroaggregates of human serum albumin. These particles lodge in the terminal arteriolocapillary bed in proportion to the regional blood supply. The same views as for the ventilation scan are then recorded so that a comparison can be made.

A current chest X-ray is required at the time the lung scan is performed to categorize the changes in the lung scan and exclude other abnormalities, such as cardiac failure, chest infection, or a tumour, which may account for the patient's symptoms.

A normal perfusion study will virtually exclude a diagnosis of pulmonary embolism. An abnormal perfusion image, with normal ventilation in the affected lung regions, and a normal chest X-ray will give a diagnosis of high probability of pulmonary embolism.

Heart scanning

Some chemotherapeutic agents are cardiotoxic. A convenient method of assessing cardiac function at intervals during treatment is to measure the left ventricular ejection fraction (LVEF). Gated blood-pool imaging is performed for this purpose. It involves taking a sequence of images showing the cardiac blood pool at different times in the cardiac cycle. The most commonly used pharmaceutical is ^{99m}Tc-labelled red blood cells. To label the red blood cells it is necessary to give an intravenous injection of stannous pyrophosphate and then 20–30 minutes later one of ^{99m}Tc pertechnetate. Data are acquired using physiological gating, using the electro-cardiogram (ECG) signal from the patient. The technique is often referred to as a multiple gated acquisition (MUGA).

Total kidney function non-imaging test

Some chemotherapeutic agents are nephrotoxic. A method of monitoring kidney function during treatment is by measuring the glomerular filtration rate (GFR). This is best estimated by using ^{51}Cr-EDTA, but ^{99m}Tc-DTPA may also be used. After intravenous injection of the radiopharmaceutical, blood samples are taken at intervals between 2 and 6 hours. GFR is calculated by measuring the clearance of the radiopharmaceutical from the blood. No urine collection is required and the preparation is simple and more reliable than creatinine clearance. This technique is suitable for use in children.

Localization of tumours

No perfect tumour-specific radiopharmaceutical has been described as yet; some however, are more specific than others.

Iodine-131

Well-differentiated thyroid tumours retain sufficient function to concentrate iodine. The ^{131}I is given orally and imaging performed 48 hours later. Whole-body imaging for the identification of metastases is of considerable value and may be repeated to assess the results of ablation therapy. It is also used to detect remnant thyroid tissue in cases where surgery has been incomplete.

M-iodobenzylguanidine

M-iodobenzylguanidine (MIBG) may be used in the localization of active catechol-amine metabolic tumours and their metastases. It has been termed a neuroendocrine tumour-seeking agent. This group of tumours includes adrenal medulla tumours (phaeochromocytoma) and neuroblastomas. The radiopharmaceutical may be labelled with either ^{123}I or [131]I.

The diagnosis of phaeochromocytoma has been made easier by the introduction of sensitive biochemical tests. However, MIBG imaging is of value in the pre-operative localization of tumour sites and in cases of suspected post-operative recurrence.

Although neuroblastoma can normally be diagnosed using X-ray CT, the uptake of MIBG can be used to provide a more specific diagnosis and for the evaluation of tumour spread, particularly to bone marrow metastases.

Octreotide

Octreotide is used in the localization of primary sites and metastases of GEP tumours (gastro-entero-pancreatic endocrine tumours). It attaches to somatostatin receptors in tissue where, as a consequence of the disease, the cell surfaces contain these receptors in a more than physiological density. However, in patients where the disease has not led to increased receptor density, imaging will not be successful. The radiopharmaceutical is labelled with indium-111.

Approximately 2% of the administered activity locates in the liver and can be excreted via the bile into the intestinal tract. Administration of a laxative is necessary in patients not suffering from diarrhoea to differentiate stationary activity accumulations in lesions in, or adjacent to, the intestinal tract, from moving accumulations in the bowel contents.

Monoclonal antibodies

Monoclonal antibodies to various tumour constituents can be labelled and used for imaging primary and metastatic sites and have potential for therapy. However, there are considerable problems with specificity and background activity in other tissues. Useful results have been obtained in gastrointestinal and ovarian tumours and melanoma, mostly using monoclonal antibodies labelled with ^{123}I or [111]In.

4

Radiotherapy: principles and practice

J D BRADSHAW and M H ROBINSON

The origins of radiotherapy date back to the 1890s, when Becquerel discovered natural radioactivity, and Roentgen discovered X-rays. Following Becquerel's discovery the Curies extracted a radiation-emitting element from pitchblende – radium.

It soon became evident that these radiations have a damaging effect on tissues, and that in some situations the damaging effect is greater for malignant tissues than for normal tissues. Before the turn of the century, the first malignant tumour (a basal cell carcinoma of the skin) had been treated successfully by irradiation.

Since the momentous work of the Curies, many more radioactive elements have been discovered or produced artificially. Some have proved of immense value as sources of radiation for treatment purposes, and many have valuable applications as diagnostic tools.

Sources of X-rays and γ-rays

X-rays are generated when electrons which have been accelerated across an evacuated tube between a heated filament (cathode) and a metal target (anode), interact with the electrons of the atoms in the target. The energy of this X-radiation is directly related to the energy of the incident electrons, which in turn is directly related to the electrical potential difference applied between the anode and cathode. For general radiotherapy the energy range is 10 kV to 8 MV; the energy of naturally occurring radiation shows marked differences from one source to another. The γ-rays from radioactive elements emanate from the nuclei of the atoms of the elements. For practical purposes, there is no difference in the properties or effects of X-rays and γ-rays of equivalent energies.

The radiation identified by Becquerel was of electromagnetic type (γ-radiation). The nuclei of radioactive elements may also emit particulate radiation, consisting of particles composed of two protons and two neutrons (helium nuclei) called α-rays, and electrons called β-rays. The β-radiation from certain elements has a place, albeit limited, in the treatment of malignant disease; α-rays are of little value in this respect.

In addition to the particulate radiation from radioactive elements, it has become possible to accelerate subatomic particles in electrical machines, and to use these particles as defined beams for treatment purposes. The first such beams were of electrons, equivalent to high-energy β-rays. More recently, it has become possible to

X-rays
Grenz rays (10–15 kV energy)
Superficial X-rays (80–140 kV)
Deep X-rays (200–300 kV energy, sometimes termed orthovoltage X-rays)
Supervoltage or megavoltage X-rays (2–20 MV and above, but usually in the range
  4–8 MV)

Radioisotopes
α-rays (of little value)
β-rays (more penetrating, and of value for superficial areas)
γ-rays
  Small sealed sources
  High-activity sources, for external beam treatment (so-called teletherapy sources)

Particulate beams of high energy
Electrons
Neutrons
Protons

Table 4.1   Radiation used in the treatment of cancer

generate beams of neutrons and of protons, and beams of other particles are being investigated.

The unit in which the dose of radiation absorbed in tissue used to be measured was the rad, which was defined as 100 ergs per gram of tissue at the point in question. With the introduction of the SI system of units, the basic unit became the Gray (Gy); 1 centiGray (cGy) is equivalent to 1 rad.

Modes of application of radiation therapy

The sources of the various radiations available have determined their chief modes of application. Beams of X-rays, and of γ-rays from small high-activity sources, can be directed from outside the body at tissue volumes in the body. Smaller radioactive sources, suitably mounted, can be applied to accessible body cavities; the best example of this technique is intracavitary treatment of a carcinoma of the uterine cervix. Radioactive elements as colloidal suspensions, or as soluble compounds in solution, have limited applications in closed body cavities, such as the pleura and peritoneum, or by direct injection into the tissues.

The forms of radiation currently available to the radiotherapist, and well established in practice, are shown in Table 4.1.

Mode of action of X-rays and γ-rays

When an X-ray or γ-ray beam passes through tissue, ionization is produced; this causes physiochemical changes in the cells of the tissue, resulting in damage to the intracellular mechanisms. Depending on the site and the degree of damage, recovery of function may or may not ensue; the cells of the tissue may survive or may die. The energy absorbed from a beam by this ionization process gradually reduces its residual energy, so that the dose delivered decreases with increasing depth of penetration.

Dose distribution in the tissues

For radiation generated at energies up to about 1 MV, the most intense ionization is in the superficial tissues; the maximum dose is on the surface. At energy above 1 MV, the most intense ionization is deep to the surface, with rapid build-up to a peak in the superficial layers and more gradual fall-off thereafter; the ionization on the surface being relatively low. For 4 MV X-rays, the so-called build-up zone is about 1 cm, for 8 MV X-rays it is about 1.75 cm, and for cobalt-60 radiation it is about 0.5 cm.

Beyond the zone of maximum dose, the energy of an X-ray or γ-ray beam is attenuated in an exponential manner, and the gradient of this absorption depends on the energy of the incident beam. For low-energy X-ray beams in the range 10–140 kV, most of the energy is absorbed in the superficial layers of the tissue, so that only very superficial volumes are treated adequately. At energies of 10–15 kV the dose delivered to the subcutaneous tissues by a beam applied directly to the skin surface is very low, and these energies of radiation have no place in the treatment of malignant conditions. In the range 60–140 kV, the depth of adequate dosage is sufficient to treat superficial skin malignancies (basal and squamous cell carcinomas of limited infiltration).

X-rays generated in the energy range 200–300 CV (orthovoltage) used to be the standard tool of the radiotherapist. Depth doses were adequate for the treatment of many malignancies, although to achieve a satisfactory total dose to a deeply situated tumour volume (e.g. carcinoma of the bladder or of the oesophagus) several convergent beams were necessary. The advent of supervoltage X-rays has made it much easier to achieve an adequate total dose from three or four incident beams.

Teletherapy γ-ray sources

The radiation from γ-ray beam units is comparable with that from supervoltage X-ray machines. The two isotopes in general use are cobalt-60 (^{60}Co) and caesium-137 (^{137}Cs). These emit radiation equivalent to about 3 MV and 600 kV X-rays, respectively. One major practical difference between the X-ray and the γ-ray units is that the radioisotopes gradually become less active, having specific half-lives for this activity. The half-life for ^{60}Co is 5.3 years; that for ^{137}Cs is 30.0 years.

Regular corrections for activity, and therefore for radiation output, have to be made, and the sources have to be replaced when the output falls to levels at which treatment exposure times become unacceptably long. The output from X-ray machines remains fairly constant at all times.

Techniques of radiation beam therapy

Beams of X-rays or γ-rays may be applied as a single direct beam, as an opposed pair of beams either tangentially to, or directly through, the tissues to be irradiated, or as multiple beams all convergent on the volume to be irradiated. For example, an accessible superficial area can be covered by a single direct beam (or field), and the energy can be relatively low, for example 100 kV for an early carcinoma of the skin. Higher energy beams, such as 4 MV X-rays or ^{60}Co γ-rays, can be used for deeper areas.

In situations requiring irradiation of larger volumes of tissue, a parallel opposed pair of beams can be used. By this arrangement, the falling dose with increasing depth of penetration from one beam is countered by the falling dose from the opposite beam. Depending on the energy of the beams, and on the thickness of the tissue section, the whole block may be fairly uniformly treated, for example using supervoltage X-rays and large fields.

Accurate application of beams

When a limited deeply situated volume is to be treated, for example a carcinoma of the middle third of the oesophagus, or a carcinoma of the bladder, multiple beams of radiation all directed at the required high-dose volume are needed. This requires precise application of beams. Surface reference points can be marked on the skin surface if the patient can be positioned easily and comfortably so that immobility can be ensured, and if the skin is not lax and therefore not easily displaced. Otherwise, some form of mould or shell to fit the region accurately is necessary; usually this is made from cellulose acetate or similar material.

Treatment simulators

Radiographs are of great value in verifying the extent and position of areas covered by radiation fields. A patient can be set up in each treatment position and the radiation from the therapy machine used to obtain the radiographs. However, all but the lowest energies used in the treatment of malignant disease produce poor quality films. Also, time which would be available for treatment exposures is used for the verifications. Therefore, units have been developed with the facility of reproducing treatment set ups and using a diagnostic X-ray tube as the source of the radiation. Good quality films can be obtained, and valuable treatment time is not lost.

Treatment verification is still an important function of treatment simulators, but their main use now is the accurate localization of the volume to be irradiated. With verification of the field positions as the final part of the simulation, CT scanning has proved of immense value in visualizing the limits of tumour volumes, and not infrequently indicates wider limits than those assessed from other investigations. Furthermore, facilities are now available for superimposing, on the images of a CT scan picture, the positions of radiation beams and the resulting dose distribution. This may lead to greater accuracy and homogeneity of the high-dose distribution in the tissues.

β-ray therapy

The term β-ray therapy is applied to the use of relatively low-energy electrons emitted by radioactive isotopes. The energies are such that the range of the electrons in the tissues is very limited, being of the order of 3–5 mm. β-ray sources can therefore be used as surface applicators or plaques to treat very superficial lesions, such as port-wine stain type haemangiomas (if in fact radiation therapy is indicated). They can also be used as surface contact solutions or collodial suspensions in body cavities, such as the pleural and peritoneal spaces, to treat effusions due to thin layers of tumour on these surfaces. In the latter applications they are termed 'unsealed sources'. Their limited depth of penetration confines their use to such superficial lesions and they are of no value in the treatment of malignant skin tumours or of bulkier tumour deposits on serous surfaces. The most common use of these is ^{131}I therapy for hyperthyroidism and thyroid cancer.

Small sealed sources

Small sealed γ-ray sources have been used since the earliest days of radiotherapy. Nowadays, ^{137}Cs and iridium-192 isotopes are most commonly used. Iridium-192 has a half life of 74 days and is used either uncovered as hairpins (single or double) or is loaded down plastic tubes inserted in the tissues around the tumour. Intracavity caesium therapy for carcinoma of the cervix and the body of the uterus is considered in Chapter 12. The advantages of using these sources compared with teletherapy machines is that they can be inserted close to the tumour and the dose from them falls off with the distance squared. In this way, the dose received by normal tissues distant from the tumour is reduced compared with external beam radiotherapy. Safety considerations have brought about the introduction of afterloading systems. In these systems, the appropriate tubes are inserted into the patient under anaesthesia. The patient is then taken to the treatment room where the tubes are connected to a machine which can be programmed to deliver caesium or iridium isotopes into the tubes for any period of time. When the patient needs nursing, the sources can be returned to the treatment safe for a short time. These systems have much greater flexibility than the old-fashioned manual loading systems.

Iridium-192 can be used to treat superficial tumours in the accessible sites, the classic example being that of a localized and superficial carcinoma of the lateral wall of the tongue. The hairpins have to be left *in situ* for approximately 6–7 days to deliver the calculated dose.

Electron beam therapy

The term electron therapy is usually applied to the use of defined beams of high-energy electrons produced in electrical machines, and applied in much the same way as single beams of X-rays or γ-rays. However, the range of electrons in the tissues is finite and is related to the energy of the incident beam.

The dose delivered in the tissues is constant within $\pm$ 10% to a depth of about two-thirds of the maximum electron range. Therefore, virtually homogeneous doses can be delivered to defined blocks of tissue to a depth determined by the energy of the beam, with little radiation dose beyond the high-dose volume.

Electron beams are of value in the treatment of some tumours, for example in the head and neck region. The useful range of energies is about 10–35 MeV; 20 MeV electrons have a treatment range of 5 cm.

Neutron beam therapy

There are theoretical reasons to believe that neutron therapy might overcome the difficulties inherent in eradicating large necrotic hypoxic tumour masses. There is evidence that this is the case, but it has become clear over recent years that late normal tissue damage is far too severe for neutron therapy to have a place in routine radiotherapy.

Proton beam therapy

Beams of high-energy protons have a limited place in radiotherapy. Protons have the same mass as neutrons, but whereas neutrons are electrically neutral, protons carry unit positive charge. Like other accelerated particles, protons have a finite maximum range in the tissues, which is dependent on the incident energy. Protons of 100 MeV energy have an average tissue range of about 10 cm. However the energy distribution along the track of a proton in the tissues is different; the energy imparted is relatively low for most of the track, but as the particle slows down the energy imparted rises rapidly. Thus, the so-called 'linear energy transfer' is highly concentrated at the end of the particle's path. This localized high intensity of ionization can be made to coincide with the tumour to be treated, provided this is small, by selecting an appropriate incident energy. It has been used, for example, in the treatment of pituitary tumours. Proton beams can be generated in cyclotrons; very high energies are required, and the beams are narrow.

Hyperbaric oxygen and radiotherapy

The amount of oxygen available to cells may be increased by increasing the oxygenation of their blood supply. Under normal conditions, the haemoglobin is almost saturated with oxygen, and the amount in the blood can only be increased by increasing the amount of oxygen in simple solution in the plasma. Breathing pure oxygen at atmospheric pressure increases the arterial oxygen content very little, but a significant rise can be achieved at a pressure of 3 atm (304 kPa). In practice, this is the maximum pressure tolerated by an unanaesthetized person.

Nevertheless, a conscious patient can be enclosed in a pressure vessel, filled with pure oxygen, and the pressure raised to three times that of the atmosphere. This technique requires repeated pressurizations, and the technical difficulties, quite apart from the psychological aspects, are great. The number of treatment exposures has to be reduced below the usual schedule of five times each week, and treatment techniques must be simplified.

Improved results have been reported from some randomized trials of hyperbaric oxygen therapy, but not from others, and the technique is not firmly established in general radiotherapy practice.

Radiosensitizers

There have been many reports of investigations into the radiosensitizing effects of so-called electron-affinic agents on hypoxic cells. These agents appear to mimic the radiobiological action of oxygen without being metabolized. They can diffuse into avascular areas.

They must be non-toxic, or midly so. They must be simple to administer, preferably by mouth, and be well absorbed. A number of agents have been investigated, including misonidazole. Unfortunately, no definite clinical benefit has been achieved and they have not yet entered routine clinical practice.

After-loading techniques

The handling of sealed sources of radiation for interstitial or intracavitary therapy exposes the operator and other staff to a relatively small but finite radiation dose. The dose depends on the activity of the sources, the distances of the sources from the individuals and the time of the exposure. The last factor depends on the dexterity of the operator and the complexity of the manoeuvres involved. With practice the time taken for procedures is reduced.

Nevertheless, any reasonably obtained reduction in the exposure of staff to irradiation is to be commended, and with this aim after-loading techniques have been developed. These require the insertion of applicator holders into the area to be treated, for example, vagina, uterine cavity, side of tongue, or tissues of the chest wall. Radio-opaque dummy sources are then inserted, and the positions checked radiologically, and modified if necessary, after which the dummy sources are replaced by active ones.

In some techniques, the insertion of the radioactive sources is done manually; in others it is done mechanically by remote control, as in the Cathetron and Selectron systems. For the latter techniques, highly active sources can be used so that insertion times are short, but this requires a specially protected room for the treatment.

Fractionation in radiotherapy

Just as normal cells of different tissues are not all equally sensitive to the damaging effects of ionizing radiation, so the cells of different tumours differ in their sensitivity to such damage. Furthermore, the sensitivity of any particular tumour cell type varies with the phase of the cell cycle at which it is irradiated. Cells are more sensitive immediately before mitosis.

The use of multiple exposures in radiotherapy is termed fractionation, and is applied to the treatment of most malignant conditions. Sometimes, a single exposure of superficial X-rays is used for a small superficial basal or squamous cell carcinoma of the skin, but the cosmetic results are inferior to those from fractionated treatment, and the risks of late tissue breakdown are greater.

Fractionated treatments may range in number from four to 25 or more, depending on the type of malignancy and the volume of tissue concerned, and on the total dose to be delivered. Usually, treatment exposures are given daily from Monday to

Friday each week. Sometimes, treatments are given three times a week on Monday, Wednesday and Friday; occasionally once weekly schedules are used.

The fractionation used in radiotherapy over the last 50 years has been pragmatic and varies between radiotherapy centres. There has been considerable interest recently in trying to determine the optimum fractionation for the treatment of a variety of conditions. Head and neck cancer has been a major target for this work. There is clear evidence that daily fractionation may not be optimal and that accelerating treatment so that it is completed over a shorter period of time or giving a higher total dose by the use of multiple daily small fractions may improve tumour control. Both these premises are being investigated and results should be available in the next few years.

Radiosensitivity of tumours

The differing degrees of sensitivity to radiation damage shown by the cells of different tumours makes it possible to divide them broadly into three groups: radiosensitive; limited sensitivity; and radioresistant. It must be stressed, however, that these terms are not absolute, there is some variation in each group, and some overlap between them. Nevertheless, the subdivisions in Table 4.2 are useful.

Radiosensitive tumours

In general, the radiosensitive tumours respond well to radiotherapy and localized disease may be cured by appropriate doses of radiation alone. In more bulky stages,

---

Radiosensitive tumours
Malignant lymphomas
Seminoma of the testis
Medulloblastoma, neuroblastoma, Wilms' tumour (nephroblastoma)

Tumours of limited sensitivity
Squamous cell and basal cell carcinomas of the skin
Carcinomas of the mouth, including tongue and lip
Carcinomas of the accessory nasal sinuses
Carcinoma of the bladder
Carcinoma of the larynx

Radioresistant tumours
Osteosarcoma
Fibrosarcoma, liposarcoma, and the myosarcomas
Malignant melanoma
Large bowel adenocarcinomas
Gliomas

Table 4.2   Examples of the radiosensitivity of tumours

for example Hodgkin's disease, localized radiotherapy may be combined with chemotherapy to optimize tumour control. Indeed, for some malignancies which have a tendency to disseminate early, cytotoxic therapy has the major role in the initial definitive treatment regimens, with greatly improved results. For example, the addition of cytotoxic therapy to surgical excision and radiotherapy for Wilm's tumour has resulted in a rise in the chance of normal life expectancy from about 30% to 90% overall. The comparable figures for Hodgkin's disease are from about 5% to 45% overall.

Tumours of limited sensitivity

The total dose of radiation tolerated by normal tissues decreases as the volume irradiated increases. Tumours of limited sensitivity are sufficiently sensitive to be curable in many cases if the volume to be irradiated is small and tolerance high, but not so if the volume is large and tolerance correspondingly lower. An example is that of an early localized tonsillar carcinoma with a curability of about 75%, compared with a more advanced local lesion with inoperable lymph node deposits in the neck, which is curable in only a few instances.

Radioresistant tumours

Tumours in the radioresistant group show some slight variations in their level of response to irradiation, but in general all would require doses in excess of local tissue tolerances to produce any significant response. Therefore they cannot be eradicated by this form of treatment; surgical excision, if possible, offers the only chance of cure. Nevertheless, some show partial responses to irradiation, and this form of treatment can offer useful palliation of otherwise untreatable malignancies in carefully selected cases. The availability of cytotoxic therapy has improved the prospects in some malignancies in this group using combined treatment regimens.

Radiation effects on normal tissues

The damaging effects of radiation are induced in normal as well as abnormal tissues. Under favourable circumstances these effects can be lethal to tumour cells and sublethal to normal cells, so that the tumour cells are killed whereas the normal cells can recover. However, all normal tissues have a level of damage beyond which recovery does not occur; this is termed the 'tolerance dose'.

Many treatment situations require the use of doses approaching the tolerance doses of normal tissues in the treatment volume, so that inevitably there will be significant damage to them. This damage is evident clinically as the 'radiation reaction' in the skin and mucous membranes within high dose volumes. The reaction follows much the same course in both skin and mucosa, first being evident between 2 and 3 weeks from the start of treatment as erythema of the skin and infection of the mucosa. Over the next 2 weeks the intensity of the reaction gradually increases. In the skin, this leads to scaling (dry desquamation) and a variable degree of pigmentation, and may progress to superficial desquamation with serous exudation (moist desquamation). In the mucosa it leads to an exudation with the formation of a fibrinous deposit (fibrinous reaction). In both situations, there is associated discomfort and soreness towards the height of the reaction. A mucosal reaction in the pharynx or oesophagus will be associated with dysphagia, in the rectum it will be associated with tenesmus and diarrhoea, and in the bladder it will be associated with frequency and dysuria.

Skin and mucosal reactions usually reach their height by the fifth week, and gradually subside thereafter over a period of 3 or 4 weeks. Relatively low doses of radiation will produce epilation. Usually this becomes evident during the third week, and hair regrowth usually commences after 2 or 3 months. Higher doses may result in permanent epilation, and certainly this is to be expected from doses approaching the tolerance of the skin. After long periods, other changes become apparent. Skin which has received full dose treatment becomes thinner and smoother, hair follicles and sweat glands become scanty, and telangiectases develop. Such skin is more liable to breakdown if damaged, even by sunlight or cold, and may be slow to heal, so-called late radiation necrosis. Late malignant change in heavily irradiated skin occurs occasionally. Mucous membranes in high dose areas also become atrophic and their natural secretions reduce; again telangiectases may develop. In subcutaneous tissues, fibrosis develops and may become marked. Other irradiated normal tissues also manifest radiation damage, but the effects are usually not so clinically obvious. However, some are very easily damaged, for example the cornea and lens of the eye, the salivary glands, the lung parenchyma, the brain and spinal cord tissues, and the renal tissues. If any of these tissues are within a volume to be irradiated, the total dose delivered must be reduced appropriately.

Healthy teeth do not show any evidence of direct radiation damage. Irradiation of the gums, however, results in some recession around the necks of the teeth which thus become exposed, and if salivary tissue is also within the high dose volume the quality of the saliva changes and this predisposes to dental caries. If there are caries in the teeth, in a volume to be treated, it is beneficial to deal with them before starting radiotherapy, unless the delay would be unacceptable.

The haemopoietic tissues of the body are also very susceptible to radiation damage. The irradiation of large volumes containing red bone marrow will result in falls in the peripheral blood leucocyte and platelet counts, and these falls may limit the total dose which can be delivered. Immunosuppression may be severe. Changes in the haemoglobin level are much less and are much slower to develop.

When large volumes are irradiated, general effects are evident in the form of so-called radiation sickness. This is a syndrome of nausea, vomiting, and general lethargy. It is related to the actual volume of tissue treated, and also to the site treated; it is more marked if the upper abdomen is within the field. Its severity is also related to the rate at which treatment is given.

Management of radiation reactions

Skin reactions

The management of skin reactions to radiation commences with the start of radiation treatment. The irradiated area should be kept dry and exposed to the air as much as possible. Local application is restricted to bland talcum powder (without added perfume or antiperspirant) unless moist desquamation develops, when a protective and mildly antiseptic application is permissible. Moist desquamation in skin near the eye can be treated with a steroid antibiotic eye ointment. Since skin which is reacting is delicate, clothing in contact with it should be soft and non-irritant.

Mucosal reactions

The management of mucosal reactions depends on the site, but a high fluid intake is vital in all cases. In the mouth, frequent bland mouthwashes (e.g. dilute sodium bicarbonate solution) are indicated from the start of radiotherapy; this helps to keep the mouth clean and free of food particles and exudate. Later, a mouthwash with mildly antiseptic effects is helpful. Not infrequently mouth reactions are complicated by monilial infections, in which case an antifungal agent is required (e.g. nystatin). Pharyngeal reactions produce dysphagia and soothing mixtures (e.g. an antacid mixture containing a topical anaesthetic) are helpful when taken before meals. In the later stages, antibiotics can be of benefit, and oxytetracyline in particular is effective.

Bladder mucosal reactions

In the management of bladder mucosal reactions, a good fluid intake and hence good urinary output is essential. The urine must be checked regularly for the presence of infection, which if detected must be appropriately treated.

Bowel reactions

Bowel reactions may lead to troublesome diarrhoea. Again, a good fluid intake is essential, together with an antidiarrhoeal preparation (e.g. kaolin and morphine mixture, or codeine phosphate) or an anti-spasmodic preparation (e.g. loperamide) given with due caution. Rectal mucosal reactions are aggravated by the presence of hard faeces, and a small dose of liquid paraffin by mouth each morning may prove very effective in softening and lubricating the lower bowel contents.

Radical or palliative treatment

In the treatment of malignant disease, it is important to determine in each case whether cure of the disease is possible or probable. If cure is likely, the inevitable side-effects and local reactions to treatment are more than justifiable. On the other hand if cure is unlikely, it is vital that treatment offers improvement in the symptoms present, without the addition or substitution of significant symptoms from the treatment itself. The probable side-effects and local reactions to treatment must be carefully weighed against the expected benefits. This applies equally well to all forms of cancer therapy.

Therapeutic aspects of nuclear medicine

The radionuclides used in therapeutic nuclear medicine invariably emit β-minus (β–) particles and it is this form of ionizing radiation which acts locally on the target organ. The radionuclides most commonly used are iodine-131, phosphorus-32, yttrium-90 and strontium-89.

Iodine-131

Thyroid cancer

Iodine-131 therapy is given for papillary or follicular carcinoma of the thyroid gland, where there is known incomplete surgical excision or metastases. In order to get iodine uptake in metastases, it is first necessary to remove all residual normal thyroid tissue either by total thyroidectomy or by giving an ablative dose of radio-iodine. After ablation, patients are given replacement thyroxine or triiodothyronine tablets.

Assessment for further therapy is carried out when the patient has been off thyroxine for at least 5 weeks or off triiodothyronine for at least 10 days. The treatment may be repeated several times if there is adequate tumour uptake.

The patient is admitted to a single room with his or her own toilet for a period of 3 days. No crockery or linen used by the patient is removed from the room until it has been monitored for radioactivity. Patients should not be pregnant or breast feeding at the time of therapy and preferably a pregnancy test should be performed.

The following radiation precaution instructions are given to patients following ^{131}I therapy depending on the retained activity at the time of the patients' discharge from hospital.

Retained activity below 150 MBq [131]I
Please obey the following instructions from date of discharge:

- You may return to work after 4 days.

- There are no restrictions on your travel movements.

- Avoid close contact with children and pregnant women for a period of 10 days.

- Avoid pregnancy or fathering a child for 12 months.

Retained activity 150–399 MBq ^{131}I

Please obey the following instructions from date of discharge:

- Do not return to work within at least 4 days.

- Limit close personal contact at home for at least 4 days.

- Avoid close contact with children and pregnant women for at least 10 days.

- Public transport can be used for journeys under 1 hour for the next 4 days, after that no restrictions.

- Avoid places of entertainment for 4 days.

- Avoid pregnancy or fathering a child for 12 months.

Thyrotoxicosis

Radioiodine therapy is indicated in patients who have relapsed after surgery or on adequate courses of antithyroid drugs, those in whom surgery is contraindicated or refused or where there is drug incompatibility.

Radioiodine therapy is effective, though the aim to destroy just enough of the hyperfunctioning gland to provide normal function for the rest of the patient's life is difficult to achieve. There is an inherent lack of precision in predicting the radiation dose to the thyroid and its effect and there is a likelihood that hypothyroidism will develop later.

Antithyroid drugs need to be withdrawn before treatment. Propranolol may be given for symptomatic relief. Clinical diagnosis must be confirmed by biochemical tests and the approximate size of the gland estimated from an image. Potentially fertile women should only be treated if pregnancy can definitely be excluded. Therapeutic activity is given orally, the amount depending on the type and size of the thyroid gland.

MIBG

^{131}I-labelled MIBG is used for the treatment of phaeochromocytoma and neuroblastoma in some centres.

Phosphorus-32

Primary polycythaemia and essential thrombocythaemia are myeloproliferative diseases in which ^{32}P (sodium phosphate) therapy is effective, particularly where venesection alone, or drug therapy, has proved ineffective. The initial activity administered is usually 185 MBq and the treatment is given on an out-patient basis by intravenous injection. Further treatments may be given at intervals if the condition relapses.

Strontium-89

Palliation of pain from extensive bony metastases from prostatic cancer may be achieved by an intravenous injection of 148 MBq ^{89}Sr (strontium chloride). Confirmation of bony metastases by bone scanning is advised prior to therapy. The treatment is contraindicated in incontinent patients.

Yttrium-90

Resistant joint effusions frequently accompany arthritis of rheumatoid, psoriatic or other origin. These effusions can be successfully treated by intra-articular ^{90}Y colloid. The ^{90}Y is injected into the joint, often the knee, so enacting a radioactive synovectomy. The usual activity administered is 185 MBq.

5

Cytotoxic chemotherapy: principles and practice

R E COLEMAN and B W HANCOCK

The great surgeon, Bilroth, first used chemotherapy, in the form of arsenic, in an attempt to cure his patients with lymphoma, but it was not until World War I that the effects of mustard gas on bone marrow cells were reported and responses of lymphoma to nitrogen mustard observed.

Many chemically related compounds were then screened and tested and in the 1940s methotrexate and other antimetabolite drugs were discovered. Since then, millions of new chemicals have been screened for anti-cancer activity but fewer than 50 are in regular clinical use. Nowadays, screening of compounds in cell culture and animal models is augmented by computer-aided drug design aimed at constructing chemicals for specific cellular targets of relevance in cancer.

Clinical trials of a potential anti-cancer drug pass through three phases. In phase I the dose schedule and toxicity of the compounds are defined. These studies are performed in patients with advanced refractory cancer. Clinical benefit is generally not expected and indeed rarely seen. In phase II the drug under test is administered to groups of patients with specific tumours to identify response. The dose and schedule defined from phase I trials is used for all patients. Generally a response rate of 20% or more is considered clinically useful.

In phase III, drugs showing promising activity are administered to a large number of patients in a comparative study against a current standard treatment. These trials are generally of randomized and, where possible, double-blind design. If phase III trials suggest the new treatment has advantages over established therapy then the drug will usually be licensed for wider use. Clinical trials may still continue as the drug is tried in various combination regimens, and alternative strategies to optimize its use are explored. These post-marketing studies are sometimes referred to as phase IV trials.

Although enormous advances have been made in the treatment of cancer with chemotherapy over the past 40 years, it is obvious that cure is unusual and largely confined to a few relatively uncommon malignancies which generally affect a young age group. The chemotherapy here is given with curative intent. The common solid cancers in middle to old age have not responded as favourably to cytotoxic chemotherapy and, even though worthwhile remissions can be obtained with relief of symptoms and sometimes apparent disappearance of tumour, the disease inevitably returns and the patient ultimately dies. In this situation the chemotherapy is given with palliative intent.

The effectiveness of chemotherapy ranges from almost always curative, as in gestational trophoblastic disease, through to rarely if ever achieving even a temporary

Curable	Highly responsive	Moderately responsive	Minimally responsive
Hodgkin's disease	SCLC	Colorectal	Pancreas
High grade NHL	Breast	Gastric	Kidney
ALL	Ovarian	Cervix	Brain
AML	Low grade NHL	Soft tissue sarcoma	Oesophagus
Testicular tumours	CML	NSCLC	Hepatobiliary
Childhood malignancies	Multiple myeloma	Head and neck	
GTD	Bone sarcomas	Bladder	
		Melanoma	
		Endometrium	
		Prostate	

Abbreviations: ALL, acute lymphoblastic leukaemia; AML, acute myeloid leukaemia; CML, chronic myeloid leukaemia; GTD, gestational trophoblastic disease; NHL, non-Hodgkin's lymphoma; NSCLC, non-small cell lung cancer; SCLC, small cell lung cancer.

Table 5.1   Responsiveness of advanced disseminated malignancy to chemotherapy

response. Table 5.1 classifies tumours according to their clinical responsiveness to cytotoxic chemotherapy.

It should be appreciated that the tumour burden in a patient with advanced malignancy is in the range of 10^9–10^{11} cells. A treatment which destroys 99.9% of a tumour from say a starting level of 10^{11} cells would reduce the tumour load to 10^8 cells, enough to make the disease disappear, but clearly insufficient for cure. Repeated cycles of treatment of this efficiency may reduce the tumour burden further, below the cure threshold, where the body's own immune mechanisms can cope with the residuum, but more typically a small proportion of resistant cells re-populate the tumour, or drug resistance develops through genetic mutation in response to repeated sub-lethal exposure to cytotoxic agents.

It follows that chemotherapy is more likely to be effective if the tumour burden is low. This is the case in adjuvant chemotherapy, given in certain clinical situations (e.g. following potentially curative surgery for breast or colon carcinoma) where there is no clinically detectable cancer left but a strong possibility of 'micro-metastases' exists, which may give rise to overt tumour recurrence if left untreated.

Administration of chemotherapy

Initially, cytotoxic drugs were given singly in relatively low doses and often continuously until tumour response was obtained. However, we now know this may promote the development of drug resistance, cause permanent damage to normal stem cells and does not take account of the rules of cell-cycle kinetics. Although this form of therapy is still appropriate for some tumours it is more usual to use pulsed

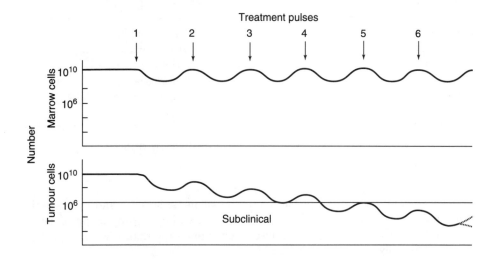

Figure 5.1 Effects of pulsed chemotherapy on tumour and bone marrow cells.

combination chemotherapy. Using cytotoxic drugs in combination gives three major advantages.

- Drugs with known effectiveness as single agents in treating a particular tumour, but with different mechanisms of action, can be used with synergistic effects.

- Drugs of different toxicities can be used to avoid cumulative adverse effects.

- Using more than one drug in a regimen may lessen the chance of resistance to the chemotherapy regimen.

Combination chemotherapy is usually given at 3–4 week intervals to allow normal tissue and bone marrow recovery. Some regrowth of the tumour population may occur, but in general, tumour repopulation is slower and less efficient than that of normal cells (Figure 5.1).

Principles of cytotoxic activity

Chemotherapy drugs are rarely, if ever, entirely selective for cancer cells and will also affect the normal cells taking part in the normal cell cycle. Cytotoxic drugs may act at different phases of the cell cycle (phase-specific), some act on the synthesis of DNA or prevent spindle formation, while others act throughout the cell cycle (cycle-specific). Most drugs, in fact, fall into the latter group and will affect cells wherever they are in the cell cycle. In general, cytotoxic drugs, unlike irradiation, will not

Cycle-specific agents	Phase-specific agents
Alkylating agents	Antimetabolites
Nitrosoureas	Vinca alkaloids
Anthracyclines	Bleomycin
Actinomycin D	Procarbazine
Mitomycin C	Etoposide
Dacarbazine	Taxanes

Table 5.2   Cycle-specific and phase-specific chemotherapy drugs

affect cells in the resting G0 phase. Examples of phase-specific and cycle-specific agents are given in Table 5.2. Clearly, tumours with a higher proportion of cells in cycle are more likely to show a response to chemotherapy than very slow growing tumours with only a small growth fraction.

The cytotoxic effects of drugs on tumour cells follow first-order kinetics, so that for a given treatment the proportion or reduction in tumour size is constant. If a tumour is chemosensitive then the number of cells will soon fall from being clinically evident (10^9–10^{12}) to clinically undetectable ($<10^8$). This is known as a complete remission, but further courses of treatment will be necessary to eradicate the tumour cell population. Whether every single cancer cell has to be destroyed by chemotherapy to effect a cure is not known. It is possible that below a certain threshold the body's immune system can cope with the remaining tumour cells.

The optimum time to stop treatment remains undefined and is largely based on intuitive or empirical decisions. Nevertheless, there are very few circumstances where continuing chemotherapy for more than six cycles seems to have any effect on either the cure rate or prognosis.

In many situations, the proportion of tumour cells in cycle is relatively small compared with the normal proliferating tissues of the bone marrow, skin and gastrointestinal tract. However, normal cells, particularly the stem cell population, are fortunately intrinsically less sensitive to chemotherapy and far more efficient at repairing drug-induced DNA damage than the cancer cells.

The time between treatments is important; if too short, the normal stem cells will not recover adequately and cumulative toxicity will result, preventing or seriously delaying further cycles. If, on the other hand, the interval between courses is too long, tumour cell recovery will be risked, allowing regrowth or the development of drug resistance to occur.

In the clinic, the appropriate time for re-treatment is judged on the blood count. If the white blood cell and platelet counts have recovered to over 3.0×10^9/l and over 100×10^9/l, respectively, full dose re-treatment can proceed. Below these levels, treatment is usually delayed or, if only marginally below these levels, the doses are reduced by 15–30%. Today, with the advent of bone marrow growth factors, it is possible to shorten the interval between chemotherapy treatments without prejudicing bone marrow stem cells. The clinical utility of this accelerated chemotherapy approach is a current area of intense investigation.

Cytotoxic drugs	Gastro-intestinal absorption	Route of excretion	Route of administration	Schedule of administration
Cyclophos-phamide	Good	Bile, urine	i.v., p.o.	Bolus
Ifosfamide	Good	Urine, bile	i.v.	Infusion
Chlorambucil	Good	Urine	p.o.	Prolonged daily
Melphalan	Good	Urine	p.o., i.v.	Few days
Carmustine	Poor	Urine	i.v.	Infusion
Methotrexate	Variable	Urine, bile	i.v., i.m., i.t.	Bolus, infusion
Fluorouracil	Variable	Urine, lungs	i.v.	Bolus, short or prolonged infusion
Mercapto-purine	Variable	Urine	p.o.	Prolonged daily
Cytarabine	Poor	Urine	i.v., i.t., s.c.	Infusion, bolus over several days
Vincristine	Poor	Bile	i.v.	Bolus
Vinblastine	Poor	Bile	i.v.	Bolus
Paclitaxel	Poor	Bile	i.v.	Infusion
Doxorubicin	None	Bile, urine	i.v.	Bolus
Epirubicin	None	Bile, urine	i.v.	Bolus
Dactinomycin	None	Bile, urine	i.v.	Bolus
Bleomycin	None	Urine	i.v., i.m., i.c.	Infusion, bolus
Cisplatin	None	Urine	i.v.	Infusion
Carboplatin	None	Urine	i.v.	Infusion
Etoposide	Variable	Urine	i.v., p.o.	Infusion or oral over several days
Procarbazine	Good	Urine	p.o.	Prolonged oral
Dacarbazine	None	Urine	i.v.	Infusion

Abbreviations: i.c., intracavitary; i.m., intramuscular; i.t., intrathecal; i.v., intravenous; p.o., by mouth; s.c., subcutaneous.

Table 5.3   Pharmacology of the most commonly used cytotoxic drugs

Pharmacology of cytotoxic drugs

As with other drugs, the absorption, distribution, metabolism and excretion of chemotherapeutic agents must be considered (Table 5.3). Absorption of oral drugs is often unreliable and certainly variable. It may be altered by the physical presence of a cancer, by changes in the patient's dietary habits and by changes in bowel motility, as well as by other drugs being simultaneously ingested. Compliance cannot be ensured, and with the exception of some alkylating agents such as chlorambucil, and low dose oral etoposide, intravenous therapy is generally preferred. In many cases, cytotoxic drugs are degraded by enzymes in the stomach and small intestine or may be intensely irritant to the intestinal mucosa.

Once in the body, hepatic and tissue metabolism, distribution into body compartments and renal excretion become relevant. The passage of drugs across the blood–brain barrier is often poor and penetration of cytotoxic therapy into large tumours with hypoxic and necrotic centres will invariably be poor. The presence of pleural or peritoneal effusions may act as an extra compartment for the distribution of some agents, notably methotrexate.

To achieve effective drug levels, the intravenous route is preferred, by either rapid injection or continuous infusion. Many drugs can now be given in the out-patient clinic by specialist nurses, and for most palliative regimens admission to hospital is no longer required.

Some drugs may be given by an intramuscular route (e.g. bleomycin) and others by subcutaneous injections (e.g. cytosine, arabinoside and asparaginase). Intracavitary instillation of drugs, such as mitomycin C may be effective for control of superficial bladder cancer, while other drugs, such as bleomycin and mustine instilled into the pleural cavity, may prevent the recurrence of pleural effusions. A few drugs are suitable for intrathecal therapy, for example methotrexate in leukaemia. However, great care must always be taken to ensure the correct dose and formulation is used because lethal side-effects may occur if these recommendations are not followed. Intra-arterial and portal vein infusion of drugs is possible and an area of continuing research. However, this form of local delivery to the tumour does not appear to have any advantage over the more straightforward intravenous route, except in the treatment of liver metastases.

For many drugs, the schedule of administration is important. Prolonged infusion of fluorouracil improves its therapeutic efficacy, while drugs such as etoposide are more effective when given in small doses over several days than when given as a large dose on a single day.

Biochemical classification of cytotoxic drugs

The most commonly used cytotoxic drugs with biochemical and kinetic classifications and usual routes of administration are shown in Figure 5.2 and Tables 5.2 and 5.3. The interaction of cancer chemotherapy agents on cancer cell proliferation can be broadly classified into five main groups: alkylating agents, antimetabolites, intercalating agents, spindle poisons, and miscellaneous drugs.

Alkylating agents

The main chemical reaction in this group of drugs is the formation of a covalent bond between highly reactive alkyl groups of the drug and the DNA double-stranded base pairs. The formation of these methyl cross-bridges either prevents the two DNA strands coming apart in mitosis or results in imperfect division with mal-union, fragmentation or clumping of chromosomes and hence cell death. Enzymes

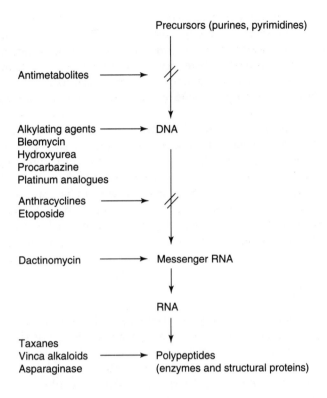

Precursors (purines, pyrimidines)

Antimetabolites

Alkylating agents → DNA
Bleomycin
Hydroxyurea
Procarbazine
Platinum analogues

Anthracyclines
Etoposide

Dactinomycin → Messenger RNA

RNA

Taxanes
Vinca alkaloids → Polypeptides
Asparaginase   (enzymes and structural proteins)

Figure 5.2   Principal sites of biochemical action of cytotoxic drugs in common use.

concerned with DNA synthesis may also be alkylated, thus preventing the formation of new DNA chains. There are a large number of drugs in this group. The properties of the more important agents are summarized below.

Nitrogen mustard (mustine) was the first cytotoxic in clinical use and is therefore of great historical interest. For many years it has been an important agent for the treatment of Hodgkin's disease. Mustine has a short half-life and is always given intravenously. Bone marrow suppression is the dose-limiting toxicity. Other side-effects are phlebitis, nausea and vomiting. Its use in Hodgkin's disease is now declining.

Cyclophosphamide requires activation in the liver for anti-tumour activity. Enzymatic hydroxylation in the liver results in the formation of active metabolites including 4-hydroxy-cyclophosphamide, aldophosphamide and phosphoramide mustard. Cyclophosphamide is one of the most widely used cytotoxic agents and is of particular value in breast cancer, lymphoma and small cell lung cancer. Bone marrow suppression is the dose-limiting toxicity. Alopecia, gastrointestinal toxicity and cystitis are other acute common side-effects.

Ifosfamide is structurally very similar to cyclophosphamide and again has valuable clinical activity in a wide range of malignancies. These include gynaecological malignancy, lung cancer, testicular tumours and sarcomas. Haemorrhagic cystitis secondary to the toxic metabolite acrolein excreted in the urine was the dose-limiting toxicity but this has largely been overcome by co-administration of the sulphydryl-containing agent mesna which reacts with acrolein before renal excretion. Bone marrow toxicity is less marked than with cyclophosphamide. Alopecia and gastrointestinal toxicity are common and some patients develop an encephalopathy characterized by lethargy, confusion and somnolence occasionally progressing to fatal coma.

Other alklylating agents include thiotepa, melphalan, busulphan, chlorambucil, treosulphan, hexamethylmelamine and the nitrosoureas BCNU (carmustine) and CCNU (lomustine). Most of these are available for administration by mouth. This, coupled with their relatively low toxicity, makes some of them particularly suited to palliative treatment in the elderly. Bone marrow toxicity is again the dose-limiting side-effect, but with the advent of bone marrow and peripheral blood stem cell support, this class of compounds particularly thiotepa, melphalan and cyclophosphamide are increasingly being incorporated into high-dose chemotherapy regimens.

Antimetabolites

These drugs inhibit DNA synthesis by interfering with the incorporation of nucleic acid bases (cytosine, thiamine, adenine and guanine). Some of these compounds closely resemble these essential metabolites and are therefore incorporated into natural metabolic pathways and enzyme systems. However, the products differ functionally from the intended products, resulting in either the inhibition of subsequent enzyme systems or in the formation of biologically inactive nuclear proteins. Cell division is therefore prevented. Each antimetabolite acts at different sites in the nucleic acid synthesis pathways.

Methotrexate is structurally very similar to, and acts as, a folic acid antagonist. Methotrexate has an affinity for dihydrofolate reductase which is a hundred times greater than folic acid and leads to inactivation of the enzyme. Dihydrofolate reductase normally reduces the inactive dihydrofolate form of folic acid to the active tetrahydrofolate form. Folic acid is essential for the transfer of methyl groups in DNA synthesis, and without the active form of folic acid the formation of purines and pyrimidines is impossible, stores of these molecules are depleted, and precursor synthesis is halted.

Methotrexate is used in the treatment of leukaemias and lymphomas and germ cell tumours. The drug is particularly effective in the treatment of persistent gestational trophoblastic disease where low doses are usually sufficient to cure this rapidly proliferating condition.

The principal side-effects are bone marrow toxicity and mucositis affecting the lips, mouth and pharynx and occasionally the small bowel. Renal toxicity occurs with higher doses of methotrexate but this can be reduced by vigorous hydration and alkalinization of the urine to restrict methotrexate crystal deposition in the renal tubules. The side-effects of methotrexate can be largely overcome by administration of leucovorin (folinic acid) 24–36 hours after administration of methotrexate. Folinic acid is in itself a tetrahydrofolate capable of restoring nucleic acid synthesis as well as displacing methotrexate from dihydrofolate reductase. Methotrexate is also taken up by pleural and ascitic fluid. Re-entry into the circulation is slow, leading to prolonged cytotoxic plasma levels and, as a result, patients in this situation are at risk of increased side-effects. Monitoring of methotrexate plasma levels is recommended when high-dose methotrexate is administered or when normal excretion of the drug cannot be guaranteed.

Analogues of pyrimidine include fluorouracil and cytarabine. The former exerts its antimitotic activity by both blocking the enzyme thymidylate synthetase and inhibiting the incorporation of uracil into RNA. Fluorouracil is rapidly metabolized making bolus administration of limited value. It is now clear that its therapeutic effect can be increased by either prolonged infusion of the drug or co-administration of folinic acid, the latter potentiating the action of fluorouracil by stabilizing the fluorouracil/thymidylate synthetase enzyme complex. Fluorouracil is most frequently used in breast cancer and gastrointestinal malignancies, particularly those arising in the colon and rectum, where it has an important role in both adjuvant therapy and the palliation of advanced disease. The side-effects are schedule dependent but include stomatitis, diarrhoea and bone marrow suppression. Oral therapy is not recommended because of unpredictable and variable absorption.

Cytarabine probably acts on DNA polymerase, an enzyme vital to the final steps of DNA strand assembly. It is used mainly in the treatment of leukaemia and some lymphomas. It has little or no activity in solid tumours, although a structurally related compound, gemcitabine, is showing promising activity in a variety of solid tumours. Side-effects include myelosuppression, gastrointestinal toxicity and, at high dose, neurotoxicity.

Purine analogues include mercaptopurine and thioguanine; they block adenine and guanine synthesis. Both agents are used in the treatment of acute leukaemia, the former principally as maintenance therapy and the latter in the induction phase. Bone marrow suppression is the principal toxicity. Hepatic toxicity may occur. Allopurinol potentiates the effect of mercaptopurine.

Intercalating agents

Like alkylating agents these drugs also form cross-strands in the DNA molecule. They bind between the base pairs, either between the two strands or within a single strand, preventing cell division and precipitating fragmentation of the DNA chains. The anthracyclines have several other cytotoxic mechanisms, including free radical formation, which cause breaks in the DNA chain and chelation of metal ions which are thought to be cytotoxic.

This class of agents includes the anthracycline antibiotics daunorubicin, doxorubicin and epirubicin and the non-anthracycline antibiotics, dactinomycin (actinomycin D), mitomycin and bleomycin.

The anthracyclines are some of the most widely used cytotoxic agents especially in the treatment of breast cancer, lymphoma, leukaemia, small cell lung cancer and sarcomas. Side-effects include bone marrow suppression, nausea and vomiting, alopecia and stomatitis. In addition, cardiotoxicity may occur. Acute rhythm disturbances are seen and, with increasing cumulative amounts of these drugs, cardiomyopathy may develop, resulting in progressive cardiac failure. This important late complication of this class of agents can be largely avoided by restricting their total dose.

The non-anthracycline antibiotic, bleomycin, is an intercalating agent which is of value in the treatment of testicular teratomas, lymphomas and squamous cell tumours. It causes little acute toxicity other than fever and hypersensitivity reactions. However, its use is limited by the development of pulmonary fibrosis. This is generally dose dependent but occasionally respiratory problems occur at relatively low doses.

Dactinomycin has been in clinical use for 40 years. Again, it acts by intercalating with DNA and inhibits RNA synthesis. It is used in a variety of paediatric tumours, testicular teratoma, gestational trophoblastic disease and soft tissue sarcomas. Myelosuppression, gastrointestinal side-effects, alopecia and skin rashes are common toxicities.

Mitomycin has both intercalating and alkylating effects on DNA. It is occasionally used in gastrointestinal and breast cancers. It is a difficult drug to use because of delayed myelosuppression, particularly affecting platelets 5–6 weeks after administration, in addition to the risk of pulmonary and renal toxicity and a microangiopathic haemolytic anaemia seen with increasing cumulative dose.

Spindle poisons

The traditional drugs in this group are the vinca alkaloids which are toxic to the microtubules of the mitotic spindle, a structure which is essential for the sorting and moving of chromosomes during mitosis. Mitosis is halted in metaphase. The vinca alkaloids include vincristine, vinblastine and vindesine.

Vincristine is the most widely used, particularly in the treatment of leukaemia and lymphomas. The drug causes little myelosuppression and may stimulate megakaryocyte maturation and increase the number of circulating platelets. Neurotoxicity is the most important side-effect with peripheral, autonomic and occasionally cranial nerve damage. Paraesthesiae and loss of tendon reflexes are the early effects which are slowly reversible. Continued treatment may lead to irreversible motor weakness, foot drop and paralysis. The autonomic neuropathy most commonly presents as constipation which may progress to a paralytic ileus. The other vinca alkaloids cause less neurotoxicity but alopecia and myelosuppression are more pronounced.

More recently, an important new drug, paclitaxel (Taxol), has been introduced. This drug is also toxic to the microtubules. Paclitaxel exerts its effect by promoting the assembly of tubulin polymers which result in the formation of excessively stable microtubule structures. This prevents the formation of normal mitotic spindles at the G2–M interface. Paclitaxel and the related taxane docetaxel (Taxotere) are very promising agents for the treatment of various solid tumours, particularly ovarian and breast cancers.

Miscellaneous drugs

This group contains an ever increasing number of agents with varying, sometimes unknown, mechanisms of action. The cytotoxic effects of platinum compounds were appreciated as the result of a chance observation nearly 30 years ago. Bacteria in culture were inhibited around platinum electrodes through which an alternating electrical current was being passed. Today, the platinum analogues cisplatin and carboplatin are perhaps the most important class of cytotoxic drugs in clinical use.

The platinum analogues react through their chloride atoms with nitrogen in guanine to form cross-links between guanine bases, both between the two strands of DNA (inter-strand) and between bases on the same chain (intra-strand). There are obvious similarities with the mechanism of action seen with alkylating agents, but the clinical effects on both cancer cells and host tissues suggest the mechanistic differences seen between the platinum and alkylating agents are of importance.

Cisplatin is the most important drug in the management of germ cell malignancies and ovarian cancer and has useful activity in lung, bladder, head and neck, stomach and cervical tumours. Cisplatin has many toxic effects including severe nausea and vomiting, neurological and renal damage. Kidney damage can be reduced by vigorous pre-hydration with several litres of normal saline and mannitol before administration, followed by further intravenous hydration for 6–12 hours after cisplatin administration. In addition, potassium and occasionally calcium supplementation may be necessary. Neurological toxicity is more difficult to prevent and may lead to premature discontinuation of treatment.

Carboplatin has a similar spectrum of activity but with considerably less renal or neurological toxicity and in many situations has now replaced cisplatin. Because complex hydration regimens are not required, carboplatin can easily be given as outpatient treatment. However, bone marrow suppression, particularly thrombocytopenia, is dose limiting and makes curative combination chemotherapy more difficult to administer. The optimum dose of carboplatin can be calculated using a formula based on renal clearance.

Etoposide is one of the semi-synthetic derivatives of podophyllotoxin. It binds to tubulin in a similar fashion to the vinca alkaloids and also inhibits topoisomerase II, an enzyme involved in maintaining the three-dimensional geometry of DNA during replication. It is now one of the most widely used cytotoxic agents with an important role in the management of lymphoma, testicular tumours and small cell lung cancer. Etoposide may be given intravenously or by the oral route. It is now clear that prolonged administration is more effective than single infusions. Intravenous administration over 3–5 days or oral therapy for 7–14 days is recommended. Bone marrow toxicity is the dose-limiting side-effect and alopecia is to be expected. Nausea and vomiting are mild.

Other agents in this miscellaneous group of drugs include dacarbazine, which has alkylating effects on DNA; procarbazine, a monoamine oxidase inhibitor used in the treatment of Hodgkin's disease; hydroxyurea, an analogue of urea with inhibitory effects on the ribonucleotide reductase enzyme system used in the treatment of chronic myeloid leukaemia; mitozantrone, an anthracenedione with structural similarities to the anthracycline antibiotics which is occasionally used as a less toxic alternative to doxorubicin in the treatment of breast cancer and lymphoma; and asparaginase, an enzyme which degrades asparagine thereby depriving malignant cells of an essential nutrient. The latter has limited activity and is currently only used in the treatment of acute leukaemia.

Drug resistance

The development of drug resistance is a complex phenomenon. The schedule of treatment may be wrong so that either regrowth of the tumour is occurring, or the exposure to a phase-specific drug is too short to affect more than a small percentage of the tumour cell population. Studies have clearly shown that prolonging the administration of agents such as fluorouracil, cytarabine and etoposide improves tumour response with no increase, and sometimes a reduction, in normal tissue toxicity.

Drug antagonism may contribute to the lack of cytotoxic effect: asparaginase and fluorouracil inhibit the action of methotrexate; and paclitaxel followed by cisplatin is more effective than the reverse schedule of administration. These observations serve to illustrate the importance of careful pharmacological and clinical testing of combination chemotherapy regimens.

True tumour resistance to cytotoxic therapy may be primary and inherent or secondary and acquired. In the former, resistance results from the heterogeneity of the tumour cell population, with some clones of cells, albeit only a minority, resistant to the effects of one or more cytotoxic drugs. The latter situation suggests that tumour cells undergo genetic mutation during treatment to become drug resistant. Again, they may only be a small minority of the total tumour cell population, but with time the resistant population of cells expands to become the dominant tumour population.

The probability of resistance within a tumour is dependent on several factors. The greater the tumour population the more likely it is that genetic mutation to a drug-resistant form will have occurred. The age of the tumour is important; resistant clones are more likely to emerge with time, owing to the inherent genetic instability of cancer cells. Rapidly dividing tumours have a shorter overall life span during which resistant mutants may appear. These theories all support the use of adjuvant chemotherapy to obtain the most favourable results because earlier use of cytotoxic treatment on a small tumour volume is less likely to be compromised by drug resistance.

The precise cellular mechanisms of drug resistance are complex and probably multiple. They include: proliferation of membrane transport pumps, which facilitate removal of drug from the cell; loss of enzymes for drug activation; increased production of a target molecule, such as dihydrofolate reductase, leading to methotrexate resistance; the development of alternative biochemical pathways; and increased DNA repair mechanisms, including expression of topoisomerases capable of restoring the three-dimensional geometry of DNA after cytotoxic damage.

Development of resistance to a specific cytotoxic drug or class of agents does not necessarily confer resistance to other drugs with a different mode of action. This is, after all, one of the fundamental rationales underlying combination chemotherapy. Nevertheless, there is a lot of cross-resistance between chemotherapy drugs and clinically it is very clear that second-line therapy will only occasionally help a patient with a potentially curable cancer, such as lymphoma or testicular teratoma. In palliative treatment, the benefits of second-line chemotherapy are marginal and often disputed.

Side-effects of chemotherapy

Some of the more important side-effects of drugs in common use are given in Table 5.4. Some side-effects, such as myelosuppression, are seen with most drugs, while others are unique to individual drugs (for example cardiotoxicity with doxorubicin and related anthracyclines). Cytotoxic chemotherapy should be given only by clinical teams familiar with its use, with the infrastructure for drug administration, and the close monitoring and assessment of patients. The drugs should be prepared by a specialized chemotherapy pharmacist using appropriate facilities to ensure inhalation and skin contact are avoided.

Before chemotherapy is given, all patients should have a full blood count performed, the chemotherapy proceeding only if bone marrow function has recovered from the previous treatment. Chemotherapy can be given in the presence of anaemia, although generally transfusion is recommended, both to make the patient feel better and to overcome the tumour hypoxia which may inhibit the efficacy of anti-cancer treatments. For certain drugs, particularly cisplatin, methotrexate and ifosfamide, renal function must also be carefully checked before administration.

Complications at the injection site

This applies particularly to drugs administered by the intravenous route. Phlebitis, with or without thrombosis, of arm veins is common but can be minimized by giving the drugs in a dilute solution, via a fast-running intravenous drip. Many chemotherapy drugs are extremely irritant if injected outside a vein. Leakage of cytotoxic drugs gives local pain and induration, which with some agents may progress to necrosis and ulceration, which is slow to heal. Extreme care must be taken during intravenous administration of chemotherapy to minimize the risk of extravasation. The safety of chemotherapy has been greatly increased by employing specialist nursing staff working in a dedicated chemotherapy administration suite. Where possible, veins on the hands or forearms should be used as their patency and integrity are easier to monitor than those in the antecubital fossa.

If extravasation is suspected, the chemotherapy injection must be stopped immediately. The infusion site is then flushed with saline through the cannula and advice obtained on how best to manage the specific drug extravasation. Ice, heat, corticosteroids and hyaluronidase are all recommended in certain situations.

Intramuscular drugs may give local pain and discomfort. This is usually temporary, provided the injection is given into a bulky muscle group. Occasionally the addition of a local anaesthetic, for example lignocaine, may be necessary. Particular care is needed in patients with thrombocytopenia requiring intramuscular injections.

Myelosuppression and immunosuppression

The patient with widespread malignant disease may have suppression of bone marrow function and the lymphoreticular system before treatment is started. Cytotoxic chemotherapy initially will worsen the situation in such cases. However, as the

Cytotoxic drugs	Alopecia	Neutropenia	Thrombocytopenia	Nausea and vomiting	Mucositis	Phlebitis	Lung damage	Skin toxicity	Neurotoxicity	Cardiac	Liver	Renal
Fluorouracil	1	2	1	1	3	0	0	1	1	1	0	0
Methotrexate	1	2	1	1	3	0	1	0	0	0	2	3
Doxorubicin	3	3	2	3	3	2	0	1	0	3	0	0
Epirubicin	3	3	2	2	2	3	0	0	0	2	0	0
Daunorubicin	3	3	2	3	2	2	0	0	0	3	0	0
Mitozantrone	2	3	2	2	2	1	0	0	0	2	0	0
Dactinomycin	3	3	2	2	2	2	0	2	0	1	0	0
Mitomycin	2	2	3	2	1	1	1	1	0	1	0	2
Bleomycin	0	1	0	0	0	0	3	3	0	0	0	0
Cisplatin	1	2	1	3	1	0	0	0	3	0	0	3
Carboplatin	1	3	3	2	1	0	0	0	1	0	0	1
Etoposide	3	3	1	1	2	1	0	0	0	0	0	0
Dacarbazine	1	2	1	3	1	2	0	0	0	0	1	0
Procarbazine	0	2	1	2	1	0	1	0	1	0	1	0
Hydroxyurea	0	2	1	1	1	0	0	1	0	0	0	0
Asparaginase	1	2	1	1	2	0	0	1	2	0	2	0
Paclitaxel	3	3	1	1	1	1	0	1	2	0	0	0
Docetaxel	3	3	1	2	1	1	2	3	1	1	0	0
Vincristine	1	1	0	0	0	1	0	1	3	1	0	0
Vinblastine	2	2	1	1	1	1	0	1	2	0	0	0
Vindesine	2	2	1	2	1	1	0	0	1	0	0	0
Cyclophosphamide	3	3	2	2	2	1	1	0	0	1	0	0
Ifosfamide	3	3	2	3	2	1	1	0	0	0	0	2
Chlorambucil	0	3	2	1	1	0	0	0	0	0	0	0
Melphalan	1	3	2	2	2	0	0	0	0	0	0	1
Nitrosoureas	1	3	2	2	1	0	1	0	0	0	0	0

Key: 0, none/unknown; 1, occasional/rare; 2, well recognized; 3, common/dose limiting.

Table 5.4 Toxicity profile of commonly used cytotoxic drugs

tumour burden decreases, there is subsequent improvement in the patient's general condition and resolution of the tumour's immunosuppressive effects. Great caution is needed to avoid the possibility of overwhelming infection; regular checking of the blood count may be indicated and any infection must be treated early and aggressively. Sensible precautions should be taken to reduce the risks of transmission of infection although full reverse-barrier nursing and sterile environments are no longer considered necessary. Most infections come from endogenous organisms, particularly the patient's own gut flora, and sensible hygiene precautions and good hand-washing are usually sufficient.

Thrombocytopenia is a less common problem with solid tumour chemotherapy but is a life-threatening toxicity of treatments for leukaemia, with haemorrhage becoming increasingly likely as the platelet count falls below $20 \times 10^9/l$. Anaemia is more of a long-term complication of myelosuppression and many patients require a blood transfusion at some time during chemotherapy.

Recently, bone marrow growth factors such as filgrastim and lenograstim (granulocyte colony stimulating factors) and molgramostim (granulocyte macrophage colony stimulating factor) have been introduced into cancer care. These natural substances stimulate the development and maturation of bone marrow progenitor cells, particularly of the white cell series. Administration of bone marrow growth factors both shortens the duration and reduces the severity of chemotherapy-induced neutropenia. This reduces the risk of severe infection and enables the delivery of high doses of chemotherapy at more frequent intervals.

In some clinical situations, bone marrow stem cells, harvested either from the bone marrow itself or from the peripheral blood after stimulation with chemotherapy and growth factors, can be collected to support the administration of high dose chemotherapy. Cells are removed from the patient, then cryopreserved until after high-dose chemotherapy, with or without whole body irradiation, has been administered. Once the drugs have been metabolized the cells are re-infused and bone marrow function returns after 7–21 days.

Anaemia, leucopenia and thrombocytopenia in the patient undergoing chemotherapy for cancer should not always be attributed to the treatment. They may also indicate a paraneoplastic effect of the tumour, or indeed bone marrow involvement by the tumour. Examination of the blood film, differential white blood cell count, and a bone marrow aspirate and trephine sample will usually give the answer.

Skin, hair and mucosal problems

As with other drugs, skin rashes of various types are not uncommon with cytotoxic drugs; if they are severe, the offending drug must be stopped. Dryness of the skin is almost invariable. Mouth ulcers are uncomfortable for the patient and are a feature particularly of severe myelosuppression and/or treatment with methotrexate and anthracyclines. Analgesia and good oral hygiene with prompt treatment of oral candidiasis are of paramount importance. Abnormal pigmentation may accompany the long-term use of certain drugs (e.g. bleomycin and busulphan), and alopecia due to damage of the hair follicles is a distressing side-effect seen with many drugs including cyclophosphamide, anthracyclines and etoposide. There is no reliable way of avoiding this, although scalp cooling may be effective with low-dose anthracyclines. It is important to warn the patient of the possibility of hair loss before treatment, reassuring them that it is always temporary, and arranging for a suitable wig.

Gastrointestinal side-effects

Nausea and vomiting are common side-effects which in the past were often difficult to control and occasionally led to poor treatment compliance. The introduction of combination anti-emetic regimens and new specific anti-emetics now enables excellent control of acute (first 24 hours) emesis with even the most toxic agents, such as cisplatin. For drugs known to be severely emetogenic, a combination of a $5HT_3$ antagonist such as granisetron or ondansetron plus a corticosteroid is recommended. For moderately emetogenic agents, traditional drugs such as metoclopramide, domperidone, haloperidol and prochlorperazine are usually sufficient.

Delayed emesis is a particular problem of treatment with cisplatin and symptoms persist for several days. The underlying mechanisms are more complex and treatments less effective. Metoclopramide and dexamethasone are the best agents currently available for this type of chemotherapy-induced emesis.

Anticipatory emesis is a conditioned response to previous unpleasant chemotherapy. It requires a different treatment approach; anxiolytics and behavioural therapy being the most widely tested.

Diarrhoea is occasionally a problem, particularly with drugs like fluorouracil, but severe toxicity to the small and large bowel is extremely uncommon and symptomatic treatment is usually very effective.

Germinal cell effects

Contraception is very important during cytotoxic chemotherapy as many of the cytotoxic drugs used are teratogenic and mutagenic. Fetal conception during cytotoxic chemotherapy may result in abortion of the embryo, or in gross congenital abnormalities of the fetus. If chemotherapy has to be given during early pregnancy, termination is usually recommended.

Infertility may occur after cytotoxic chemotherapy. It is particularly a feature of high-dose alkylating agents. In women, this is accompanied by an early menopause, while in men, although sperm production is ablated, endocrine function is generally preserved. Infertility is most likely in those treated during puberty and in older patients, particularly women nearing the menopause. For men, sperm storage is now available in most centres. However, cryopreservation of ova or ovaries is not generally available. Recovery of germinal epithelium is often slow and fertility may not return for months or even years after completing chemotherapy.

If fertility is at all a possibility, the patient should be advised to avoid conception for at least a year after completion of chemotherapy. To date, the children conceived by parents who have had previous chemotherapy have shown no evidence of increased congenital abnormalities or subsequent malignant disease.

Less frequent side-effects

Cardiomyopathy, or overt heart failure, is a dose-related adverse effect of anthracycline treatment. It is more likely in patients who also receive cardiac irradiation or in those with a past history of cardiac disease. As the dose of anthracycline increases, monitoring of ventricular function by echocardiography or radionuclide angiography is recommended.

Occasionally, chemotherapy will cause lung damage. Diffuse alveolar damage, which may progress to fatal pulmonary fibrosis, is seen with high doses of bleomycin. The total dose of bleomycin should be limited and great care taken when anaesthetizing patients who have previously been exposed to this drug. Mitomycin, busulphan and certain other alkylating agents also occasionally cause respiratory problems.

Hepatotoxicity is an occasional side-effect. It usually takes the form of hepatocellular damage and may manifest as disordered liver function tests or jaundice. Long-term exposure to methotrexate is the best described cause. In addition veno-occlusive disease of the liver may accompany high-dose intensive chemotherapy.

Nephrotoxicity is a common complication of treatment with cisplatin, and great care must be taken to ensure adequate hydration of patients during cisplatin therapy. Some degree of tubular damage is almost inevitable with loss of magnesium, calcium and potassium. Tubular damage may also be seen after treatment with methotrexate or ifosfamide. Methotrexate-induced renal damage is reduced by alkalinization of the urine, while careful intravenous hydration and co-administration of mesna reduces the risk of ifosfamide-induced damage.

Neurotoxicity (which may affect peripheral, autonomic and cranial nerves) is most commonly seen with the vinca alkaloids, particularly vincristine and cisplatin. Ototoxicity is another important toxicity of cisplatin affecting particularly the appreciation of high frequency tones.

Special precautions

Drug doses are usually based on the surface area of the patient. In patients with impaired renal or hepatic function the doses of certain drugs excreted by the kidney or metabolized and excreted by the liver will have to be reduced. This information must always be checked in the relevant drug data sheet.

Interactions are a common problem with all forms of drug therapy and cytotoxic chemotherapy is no exception. Drug absorption may be affected by altering gastric emptying, for example with anti-emetics, or by changing gut flora with antibiotics. Protein-binding cytotoxics (e.g. methotrexate) may be altered by the administration of displacing drugs, such as aspirin or anti-inflammatory drugs. Allopurinol enhances the effect of mercaptopurine by inhibiting enzymes concerned with its breakdown.

During chemotherapy, the patient's quality of life is of great importance. Delivery of chemotherapy by experienced personnel in pleasant surroundings with attention to side-effects will reduce the unpleasantness of treatment to a minimum. Positive reassurance and morale boosting are also important components of the patient's treatment. It may be possible for a patient to continue working during a course of chemotherapy. In general, out-patient treatment is preferable, except for the elderly or infirm patient and in those who have to travel a long distance for treatment, when overnight accommodation may be more appropriate.

6

Other treatments

B W HANCOCK, M H ROBINSON and R C REES

The first therapeutic attempt is always the best, and sometimes the only, opportunity for cure of malignant disease. It is of the utmost importance, therefore, that the initial treatment is carefully considered. The known or likely extent of the disease, its expected response to the forms of treatment available, and its expected long-term behaviour all warrant assessment.

It may be that surgery alone, or combined with radiotherapy and/or cytotoxic chemotherapy, offers the best chance of eradication of the disease. For some malignancies, particularly those in the 'radioresistant' group, surgery is usually the only form of radical treatment available; though with the development of new cytotoxic agents and regimens, these are becoming more important in the overall management of the disease.

Surgery

Surgery is the oldest method of treating malignant disease, but only in the twentieth century has it become safe and effective with the greater appreciation of anatomical and physiological principles, the development of aseptic rather than antiseptic procedures, and the use of greatly improved anaesthetic agents and techniques.

Radical surgery

Radical surgery may result in little deformity or dysfunction alternatively significant physical and functional impairment may ensue. All surgical procedures carry some risk of operative morbidity and mortality, and in situations where a choice of treatments is available these must be carefully assessed. The general physical and medical state of the patient is also highly relevant to the form of management selected.

Tumour resection *en bloc* may offer the best opportunity for cure, where this is feasible without unacceptable morbidity or mortality. It may include removal of the regional lymphatic glands (block dissection) if these contain demonstrable deposits or there is a high risk of involvement.

Some radical surgical procedures, such as radical mastectomy for early breast cancer, have been demonstrated to be unnecessary in the majority of patients. Its use was based on the theory that breast cancer was a locoregional disease rather than a systemic one. In many women it has been supplanted by wide local excision and the use of post-operative radiotherapy. Simple mastectomy is another alternative. Radical mastectomy resulted in lymphoedema of the upper limb in a significant number of cases. The operation is associated with the name of Halstead.

Radical surgery for carcinoma of the uterine cervix was established by Wertheim. This operation involves removal of the uterus, a cuff of vagina, the fallopian tubes and ovaries, the broad ligament and the pelvic lymph glands and lymphatics. This cannot be achieved entirely *en bloc* because of the need to dissect out and preserve the ureters.

Abdominoperineal resection of the rectum for adenocarcinoma is also well established as a radical procedure. The involved section of bowel, with a generous margin proximally, and the associated mesentery and lymph glands are removed up to the level of the inferior mesenteric artery. Partial colectomy with removal of the mesentery and the lymph glands draining the affected segment is a standard operation for colonic cancer.

For operable gastric carcinoma, total gastrectomy with removal of the draining lymph glands, is undertaken. In selected cases of thyroid cancer, total thyroidectomy is appropriate. For operable involved lymph glands in one side of the neck from an ipsilateral primary tumour in the mouth area, *en bloc* dissection of the lymph glands, lymphatic channels, internal jugular vein and sternomastoid muscle offers a chance of cure.

Operative dissemination

Radical surgery for a localized tumour may not always prove curative. At operation, tumour cells may be shed into the veins or lymphatic channels, and may disseminate to produce distant metastases, or may be seeded into the wound, producing implantation deposits. Not all such cells survive, however; studies of venous blood and lymph draining from operation sites have shown the presence of tumour cells in up to 25% of cases, yet the incidence of overt metastases is much lower than this, and many of these cells must therefore be non-viable.

Adjuvant surgery

In situations where surgery alone is not potentially curative, it may nevertheless play a useful part in the management of the disease. Planned removal of a large primary tumour as a preliminary to radiotherapy and/or cytotoxic chemotherapy may be of great benefit by reducing the bulk of tumour to be treated. Clear examples of this are seen in head and neck cancer where advanced lesions of the laryngopharynx require radical surgery, which alone has a very small probability of curing the patient. Adjuvant radiotherapy is often used to eradicate residual microscopic disease in this situation.

Removal of slow growing and apparently solitary pulmonary metastases, for example from osteosarcoma or renal adenocarcinoma, may lead to an increased period of symptom-free survival.

Palliative surgery

Surgery can be of great value as palliation alone. A colostomy for lower large bowel obstruction from an advanced tumour may result in immediate relief of distressing symptoms. A tracheostomy for laryngeal obstruction may avert rapid death from asphyxia. A bypass operation for internal hydrocephalus caused by cerebral tumour may provide rapid relief of severe headaches, nausea and vomiting.

Diagnostic surgery

Diagnostic surgery is frequently of help in obtaining tumour tissue for histological diagnosis. This may take the form of a simple operation, such as an excision of a lymph node, or a more major procedure.

Other surgical procedures

The surgical management of tumours in specific sites is considered in more detail in the appropriate sections.

Immunotherapy

During the past 20 years several approaches to immunotherapy of cancer have been adopted (Table 6.1). Initially this took the form of using crude tumour cell vaccines

Passive	Administration of antibodies
Active	
Non-specific	
BCG	
C. parvum	
Levamisole	
Thymosin	
Specific	
Irradiated tumour cells	
Transfer factor	
Adoptive	
Non-specific	
Unsensitized lymphoid cells	
Specific	
Sensitized lymphoid cells	
Local	Injection into tumour (e.g. BCG)

Table 6.1   Immunotherapy in cancer

for immunization, in an attempt to promote host immunity, but on a background of host immune suppression. Further attempts to potentiate the level of immuno-competence of cancer patients using BCG, *Corynebacterium parvum*, and lev-amisole met with variable success. It is now apparent that in most instances the administration of BCG and other immunomodulatory agents, with or without autologous tumour cells, failed to induce tumour regression or potentiate anti-tumour immunity. As discussed in Chapter 1, the identification of human tumour-associated antigens (MAGE, Melan-A, gp-100, tyrosinase) which promote CTL activity has opened up new possibilities for cancer therapy. Experimentally, the CTL response is essential for tumour regression and the induction of 'solid host im-munity'. We are therefore presented for the first time with defined 'human tumour antigens', which are known to induce CTL activity, which *in vitro* at least, mediates the killing of cancer cells. More importantly, it has been shown that specific peptide sequences from each tumour antigen induce peptide-specific CTL activity, and this provides us with the opportunity to develop human tumour vaccines. At the present time, at least three peptide-based vaccines are in phase I clinical trials, and within the next few years many more will be developed. The antigens so far discovered appear to be involved in normal cell differentiation processes and therefore act as weak immunogens. It is likely that the immune system has developed a tolerance to these antigens, and strong CTL activity will not occur naturally. In order to break this tolerance and potentiate CTL activity it is proposed to use immunological adjuvants together with specific peptides for immunization. Whether this approach can be successfully applied in the clinic remains to be established. Additionally, such vaccines may have greater potential if they are used in combination with cytokine therapy aimed at restoring immunocompetence (see below).

Cytokine-based immunotherapy of cancer

As discussed in Chapter 1, cancer patients are in the main immunosuppressed and have low and sometimes negligible anti-tumour lymphocyte-mediated activity against either established cancer cells lines, or against autologous tumour cells. Several approaches, using cytokine therapy, have been shown to potentiate anti-cancer immune reactivity, and experimentally (in animal models) it is possible to cause tumour regression of both primary and disseminated disease. In particular IL-2 has been shown to boost NK cell and T cell reactivity and mediate tumour regression. In human cancer trials, IL-2 is effective in a minority of patients with secondary malignant melanoma or renal cell carcinoma. Approximately 20–30% of patients with these malignancies show either complete regression or partial regression of their tumours. The boosting *in vitro* of lymphocyte activity from individual cancer patients with IL-2 increases non-MHC restricted effector function, known as lymphokine activated killer (LAK) activity. In the main, this activity is mediated by NK cells together with a minority population of activated T lym-phocytes, however, re-infusion of cells together with IL-2 has not demonstrated a significant clinical advantage over IL-2 therapy alone. IL-2 is currently licensed for use with renal cell carcinoma and administration of this cytokine in patients with minimal residual disease has proved more effective than in patients with widespread

Treatment	Tumour type
Interferon-α	Hairy cell leukaemia
Interleukin-2	Malignant melanoma, renal cell carcinoma
Tumour necrosis factor α	Perfusion of isolated limbs (e.g. melanoma)
BCG	Bladder cancer (intravesical infusion)

Table 6.2   Biological therapy in human cancer

disease. Patient selection is important when using IL-2 therapeutically. Studies have shown that tumour regression, induced as a result of IL-2 therapy, is associated with CD8$^+$ T lymphocyte infiltration, and although the precise mechanism of regression is not fully understood it is likely that CTL activity is operative against the patients' tumour cells and causes, either directly or indirectly, tumour destruction. It is unclear at present whether this activity is specifically directed towards the recently identified human tumour antigens (e.g. MAGE encoded antigens) and further investigations are required to establish the mechanism responsible.

Other cytokines have proved of value in the treatment of certain malignancies (Table 6.2). For example, IFN-α is effective in the treatment of patients with hairy cell leukaemia (causing tumour regression in 70% of cases) probably as a result of its anti-proliferative effect. Also, the perfusion of TNF-α into limbs of patients with localized, malignant melanoma causes the complete regression of malignant foci. The use of TNF-α systemically would have lethal widespread effects, but high concentrations used locally have a direct toxic action on cancer cells. A newly discovered cytokine, IL-12, has been shown experimentally in mice to have potent anti-tumour activity. IL-12 is effective at low doses and is capable of acting synergistically with low-dose IL-2 to promote anti-tumour immunity, without inducing toxic side-effects. The use of this cytokine, either singly or in combination with other cytokines, may prove beneficial in the treatment of human malignant disease, causing an upregulation of natural immunity and antigen-specific CTL. Trials with IL-12 have recently begun and the results are keenly awaited.

At the present time we are faced with a number of options for implementing cancer immunotherapy in the clinical setting. Many of these applications are experimental, and involve the use of both cytokine-based therapy and vaccination procedures with tumour antigens or peptides derived from tumour antigens with or without immunological adjuvants. It is interesting to note that although BCG proved to be on the whole ineffective in the treatment of several human cancers, its use in the treatment of localized bladder carcinoma can cause the complete or partial regression of tumours, probably because it activates the local immune defence system. The continuing investigations in this field have revealed immunotherapies which work in specific situations. A logically and scientifically based approach to implement these treatments is required, and at each stage of the therapy, monitoring of immune responses is essential if we are to understand the mechanisms involved, and as a result develop and improve immunotherapeutic strategies.

Gene therapy

As we saw in Chapter 1, cancer is now accepted to be a genetic-based disorder. The recognition of cancer-associated genes (including oncogenes and tumour-suppressor genes) has led to 'gene therapy' becoming a reality. Theoretical manoeuvres include:

- delivering suicide genes
- transferring wild-type tumour-suppressor genes
- inhibiting oncogenes
- promoting a systemic anti-tumour response.

Endocrine therapy

The Scottish surgeon, Beatson, demonstrated in 1896 that oophorectomy can cause regression of metastatic breast carcinoma. It has since become apparent that the growth of some tumours is hormone dependent and that changing the balance of the hormonal environment can lead to regression of such tumours. A summary of the various endocrine procedures used in cancer therapy is given in Table 6.3 and some of the side-effects are listed in Table 6.4. Their more precise role is defined in the appropriate chapters on treatment.

Hormone therapy is rarely curative however, and often needs to be combined with other treatment, such as surgery, radiotherapy and chemotherapy. The recognition of the presence of hormonal receptors, particularly in breast cancer tissue, has

Tumour	Therapy
Breast	
Pre-menopausal	Oophorectomy (adrenalectomy, hypophysectomy)
Peri-menopausal	Androgens
	Corticosteroids
	Anti-oestrogens
Post-menopausal	Oestrogens
	Anti-oestrogens
	Progestogens
Prostate	Oestrogens, orchidectomy
Uterine body	Progestogens
Kidney	Progestogens
Haematological	Corticosteroids
Thyroid	Thyroxine

Table 6.3   Examples of endocrine therapy for cancer

Oestrogens
  Nausea
  Fluid retention
  Vaginal bleeding
  Feminization
  Hypercalcaemia
Androgens
  Virilization
  Cholestatic jaundice
Anti-oestrogens
  Nausea
  Skin rash
Progestogens
  Fluid retention
  Nausea
Corticosteroids
  Fluid retention
  Hypertension
  Diabetes
  Osteoporosis
  Cushingoid features
  Immunosuppression

Table 6.4   Side-effects of endocrine therapy

made the use of endocrine treatment far less empirical, since detection of these receptors appears to be a reliable method of predicting hormonal responsiveness.

The role of steroids in cancer treatment deserves special consideration. Apart from their direct cytotoxic effect they have a role in the management of certain peripheral cancer effects. The physical and psychological well-being of a patient may be transiently improved, and hypercalcaemia (in appropriate tumours) and cerebral oedema (in association with brain metastases) may respond dramatically to prednisolone and dexamethasone, respectively.

7

Cancer of the lung and mediastinum

B W HANCOCK and J D BRADSHAW

Primary lung cancer is essentially carcinoma of the bronchus. Occasionally carcinomas arise in the trachea, and malignant tumours of the pleura also occur.

Carcinoma of the bronchus

The bronchial tree is the most common single site of cancer in man. The incidence has increased since 1945. The number of deaths in England and Wales caused by bronchial carcinoma increased five-fold between 1945 and 1980. In 1945 there were 7000 deaths, in 1965 the figure was 27 000 and in 1980 there were 35 000 deaths. However, in 1985 there were 34 000 deaths, about the same number as in 1980, so the numbers may be levelling out.

The incidence is higher in men than in women in the ratio of about 4 to 1. However, this difference is decreasing, as the incidence in women increases more rapidly than in men; in fact, in men the incidence has perhaps even decreased slightly. Carcinoma of the bronchus is rare below the age of 25 years; the highest incidence is in the sixth and seventh decades of life.

Lung cancer has been recognized as an industrial hazard for many years. Inhalation of asbestos dust is associated with pleural mesothelioma and bronchial carcinoma. Dust containing arsenicals, chromates and dichromates has a similar effect on the bronchial mucosa. Atmospheric pollution from industry and the internal combustion engine contribute. The main cause, however, is smoking tobacco, particularly cigarettes.

Histology

The most common histological types of bronchial cancer are shown in Table 7.1. Over three-quarters of carcinomas arise in the main bronchi or their first divisions, and most are therefore in the hilar regions. They may be mainly intrabronchial (papilliferous) or may infiltrate the bronchial wall; most ultimately show both features and cause obstruction of the lumen. Primary bronchial carcinoma is rarely bilateral.

Local spread is to adjacent structures, such as the chest wall, mediastinum, pericardium, pleura and diaphragm. Lymphatic spread is via the mucosal, peribronchial,

Common types

- Squamous cell carcinoma (40–60% of lung cancers) arising on areas of squamous metaplasia resulting from chronic irritation and the effects of carcinogens; much more common in men
- Undifferentiated carcinoma (about 30% of lung cancers) mainly small cell (oat cell) tumours, but a few large cell lesions; more common in men
- Adenocarcinoma (about 15% of lung cancers) of equal incidence in the sexes

Less common types

- Cylindroma, which may involve the lower end of the trachea, and may be locally invasive
- Alveolar cell carcinoma, which arises peripherally in the lung
- Bronchial adenoma, usually benign
- Carcinoid tumour, usually benign

Table 7.1   Histological types of bronchial cancer

pleural and perivascular vessels, with metastases to the hilar, subcarinal, tracheo-bronchial, paratracheal and supraclavicular nodes. Blood spread most commonly results in metastases to the bones, brain, liver, suprarenal glands, kidney and the opposite lung. Spread by bronchial aspiration has also been suggested.

Clinical features

The common symptoms are cough, dyspnoea and haemoptysis, similar to those of bronchitis and bronchiectasis. Occasionally anorexia, fatigue, or pyrexia of unknown origin are the presenting features. Some patients present with superior vena cava obstruction. Hoarseness, due to left recurrent nerve palsy, or dysphagia due to pressure on the oesophagus from enlarged mediastinal nodes may develop.

Horner's syndrome (ptosis, myosis, enophthalmos and anhydrosis, on one side) results from sympathetic ganglion involvement in the lower neck. Tumours arising at the lung apex can invade the chest wall including the ribs and branches of the brachial plexus, causing Pancoast's syndrome, that is Horner's syndrome together with pain in the upper limb, wasting of the small muscles of the hand and destructive areas in the upper two or three ribs, on the affected side.

Hypertrophic pulmonary osteoarthropathy (HPOA) and digital clubbing may occur as paraneoplastic manifestations. HPOA presents as painful expansion of the lower ends of the radii and sometimes of the tibiae. Clubbing occurring without HPOA is a suggestive but not diagnostic feature.

Other non-metastatic effects include cerebellar ataxia, peripheral neuropathy, and ectopic hormone secretion (see Chapter 16). In disseminated disease there may be symptoms related to metastases.

Investigations

In the investigation of bronchial cancer, radiology is of great value. Postero-anterior (PA) and lateral films of the chest are required, since some significant parts of the lungs cannot be clearly visualized on PA films alone. Histological diagnosis is mandatory; sometimes this is established from sputum cytology but more often fibreoptic bronchoscopy, or sometimes mediastinoscopy, with biopsy is needed. In certain cases CT is proving of great value.

Treatment

It is generally accepted that the only potentially curative treatment of localized squamous carcinoma and adenocarcinoma is surgical excision, either lobectomy or pneumonectomy as appropriate. This is possible in only a small proportion of cases. In the remainder, the disease is too advanced or surgery is contraindicated by the patient's general condition, limited pulmonary reserve or coincidental disease. Radical radiotherapy is applicable only to tumours which are surgically operable, but where surgery is contraindicated on the above grounds.

Surgery is not appropriate in the management of undifferentiated small cell carcinomas (oat cell carcinomas). These tumours spread early to local lymph nodes, and disseminate early via the bloodstream, typically producing metastases in the brain, bones and liver. Chemotherapy, though only of palliative value in the majority of cases, is sufficiently active to make it the first choice in treatment. Doxorubicin, etoposide and cyclophosphamide are the three most popular agents used, often in combination. Newer agents being studied in combination chemotherapy include ifosfamide (with mesna), and cisplatin. In addition, local and cranial irradiation may be given.

For all types of lung cancer, palliative irradiation may be very helpful in the treatment of superior vena cava obstruction, haemoptysis, dyspnoea due to lobar or lung collapse, and persistent cough. It is of less value in the treatment of mediastinal pain and oesophageal obstruction. Local treatment to bony metastases usually offers good pain relief. Brain irradiation for metastases is of value only for oat cell carcinoma deposits. In the palliative treament of non-small cell carcinomas, chemotherapy may be of some value, but at present should only be given in the context of clinical trials.

The management of locally advanced but asymptomatic disease is debatable. Some authorities argue that treatment is essentially palliative and that if there are no symptoms to palliate no treatment is required. Others argue that locally advanced disease will progress and produce symptoms sooner or later and that treatment to a small volume will be more effective than to a larger volume. In practice, each case must be considered individually.

Results

The results of treatment of lung cancer are very poor. About 80% of patients die within 1 year, and the overall 5-year survival is about 5%. Pneumonectomy yields figures of about 25% at 5 years; operative mortality is 5–10%. Lobectomy gives about 30% 5-year survival, with operative mortality of 2–5%. Five-year survival for small peripheral tumours is 30%. Radical radiotherapy shows 5-year survival in a mere 3–5% of cases.

In limited-stage small cell lung cancer, chemotherapy improves survival prospects from 6 months to over 12 months; 20% will be alive and disease free after 2 years. However, late relapse will occur and by 4 years survival is reduced to about 5%. For more extensive small cell carcinoma, median survival may be prolonged from a few weeks to a few months.

Cancer of the trachea

Cancer of the trachea is rare. One series reported five cases over a 5-year period, during which 1600 cases of bronchial carcinoma were treated. It is most common in the middle and lower thirds of the trachea. Most tumours are squamous cell carcinomas; occasionally cylindromas are reported. Radical surgery is rarely possible, and radiotherapy yields poor results.

The rarity of cancer of the trachea is interesting, considering its relatively high incidence in the larynx and very high incidence in the bronchi.

Tumours of the pleura

Primary tumours of the pleura are uncommon. Most frequent are localized fibromas, which are resectable, and diffuse endotheliomas (mesotheliomas) some of which are malignant, and which may be difficult to resect and treat. In the latter tumours, local palliative radiotherapy may be needed for pain relief. Cytotoxic chemotherapy is of little value. Results of treatment are poor.

Mediastinal tumours

Primary tumours of the mediastinum are uncommon; about one-third are malignant. They are listed in Table 7.2.

Dermoid cysts

Dermoid cysts (teratomas) occur predominantly in the 10–30 year age group. Almost invariably they arise in the anterior mediastinum, usually in front of the pericardium and great vessels. Usually they contain tissues from all three layers

---

Dermoid cysts (teratomas), the most common

Neurogenic tumours
Neuroblastoma, ganglioneuroma, phaeochromocytoma arise from nerve cells of the sympathetic system
Neurilemmoma, neurosarcoma, neurofibroma arise from nerve sheaths

Thymoma

Rare tumours
Examples are: lipoma and liposarcoma; paraganglioma; haemangioma; tumours similar histologically to choriocarcinoma; benign and malignant mesenchymal tumours of the heart; mesothelioma of the pericardium (usually malignant); and leiomyosarcoma of the great vessels

---

Table 7.2   Mediastinal tumours

of the embryo, mainly skin, hair, sebaceous material and glandular tissue. Most are benign, but a few are malignant most commonly in their squamous epithelial elements.

Neurogenic tumours

Neurogenic tumours usually arise in the posterior mediastinum. They can vary greatly in size, and can weigh as much as 1 kg. If they arise from nerve elements near an intervertebral foramen the typical dumb-bell tumour results, with part inside the spinal canal and part outside. Enlargement of the foramen can be seen radiologically. The best example of this is in multiple neurofibromatosis (von Recklinghausen's disease).

Neuroblastomas occur almost exclusively in childhood. Some show areas of well-differentiated ganglioneuroma, and have a better prognosis. Occasionally, spontaneous transformation from neuroblastoma to ganglioneuroma occurs (see Chapter 15).

Thymoma

Thymomas account for about 10% of mediastinal tumours. Almost invariably they arise in the anterior mediastinum. They may be true neoplasms or simple hypertrophy of the thymic tissues. They are most common in middle age. About 10% are benign cysts; about 30% are invasive. Four histological types are described: lymphocytic, epithelial, mixed and spindle-celled. Occasionally the histological appearance resembles seminoma, and occasionally there is a granulomatous appearance which is now regarded as thymic Hodgkin's disease. Some are associated with myasthenia gravis; 10% of patients with this condition have a thymoma, and 50% of patients with a thymoma have myasthenia gravis.

Management

Thoracotomy should be considered for diagnosis and if possible for removal of the tumour. Operative mortality, in competent hands, is surprisingly low. Radiotherapy may be indicated for the primary tumour or for the residue after surgery. It may be curative in neuroblastoma and thymoma, and it may achieve long-term control in malignant teratoma. Combination cytotoxic chemotherapy is given for more widespread neuroblastoma.

Results

The results of treatment depend on the type of tumour. Benign tumours can usually be excised and do well. Thymomas vary in their response, but overall 5-year survival of 20% is reported for malignant types. For neuroblastoma the prognosis for localized tumours is good, but for metastatic disease long-term survival is less than 10%. For other tumours, the numbers treated are too small to allow for accurate assessment.

Other mediastinal tumours

Malignant lymphatic involvement is the most common cause of mediastinal tumour; malignant lymphoma and secondary carcinoma (e.g. from bronchus) are the usual offenders. The management of these tumours is discussed under the appropriate headings.

8

Breast cancer

R E COLEMAN

The breast is the most common site of malignant disease in women and the average woman has a 1 in 12 lifetime risk of developing the disease. In the UK there are over 25 000 new cases of breast cancer and about 15 000 deaths caused by it each year. The incidence of the disease increases with age; it is uncommon below the age of 30, rising steadily through the age range with the exception of a slight reduction in incidence in the early fifties just after the menopause. For women in the age group 40–44, breast cancer is the most common cause of death. Perhaps more than any other cancer, carcinoma of the breast displays an extraordinarily variable clinical course. Recurrence of the disease can be seen many years and even decades after primary treatment. Advanced breast cancer may be rapidly progressive despite all forms of treatment over a matter of a few months, or may not cause death for many years.

Aetiology

There are a number of aetiological factors which predispose to breast cancer (Table 8.1) but their precise contribution to the disease is not known. Breast cancer is essentially a disease of the Western world and is more common in women who

Definite	Probable	Possible
Increasing age	High-fat diet	Alcohol
Positive family history	Exogenous oestrogens	Viruses
Exposure to radiation		Smoking
Early menarche		Caffeine
Late menopause		
Late or no pregnancy		
Never breast fed		
Obesity		
Proliferative benign breast disease		

Table 8.1 Factors that predispose to breast cancer

experience an early menarche, late menopause, and have either never been pregnant or had their first child after the age of 30 years. Normal breast feeding is protective, while being overweight is a risk factor for breast cancer due principally to the excess conversion of androgens to oestrogens in peripheral fat. Long-term (>5 years) exposure to exogenous oestrogens, as in the contraceptive pill or hormone replacement therapy, slightly increases the risk of developing breast cancer. However, this excess risk is outweighed by the benefits of oestrogens on other organs, except perhaps in those already at high risk for breast cancer due to a strong family history of the disease. Certain types of proliferative benign breast disease predispose to cancer. A diet high in animal fat seems to be a causative factor, although dietary intervention studies have failed to show an impact on the development of breast cancer.

A positive family history is of major significance, particularly when cancer has occurred in one or more first-degree relatives and especially if this was at a young age or involved both breasts. Several important genes involved in familial breast and ovarian cancer have been identified including BRCA, which is located on the long arm (q) of chromosome 17. Despite the importance of these findings and the potential for genetic screening, only 5–10% of all women who develop the disease have one of these cancer family syndromes.

Pathology

The majority of breast cancers arise from cells lining the ducts of the breast (ductal carcinoma). In about 15% of cases the carcinoma is of lobular type while the special types of breast cancer (medullary, tubular, papillary) occur in only a very small proportion of cases. Similarly, sarcomas, lymphoma and metastatic carcinoma are unusual compared with primary epithelial tumours.

Pathological distinction between *in situ* disease and infiltrating carcinoma is of major importance in planning treatment. *In situ* disease is a locally curable condition whereas infiltrating carcinoma is often a systemic disease at the time of presentation. Infiltrating ductal carcinoma can be further sub-classified according to histological grade into good, intermediate and poor prognostic groups.

Breast cancer spreads by local infiltration into the skin and chest wall, by lymphatic spread to regional lymph nodes (axillary, supraclavicular fossa and internal mammary) and via the bloodstream to any distant organ, in particular the bones, lungs, liver and brain. Cancer in the opposite breast can develop either as a new primary or a metastasis, a distinction which can be difficult to make histologically.

Screening

Screening for breast cancer is now established throughout the UK for women in the 50–65 year age range in whom bilateral mammography is recommended every

3 years. The introduction of routine breast screening has led to the development of dedicated screening clinics with radiological, surgical and pathological input for rapid diagnosis. Screening has led to an increase in the detection of small tumours, *in situ* lesions and those of special histological type. It is now established that when screening mammography is performed as recommended and with high quality techniques the mortality from breast cancer can be reduced by 30%.

Within the next few years molecular and genetic screening is likely to develop and be relevant particularly to those with a positive family history.

Clinical presentation

Typically, a woman presents after identifying a lump in the breast. It is important to appreciate that only 10% of all breast lumps presenting to a GP will prove to be malignant. Features suggestive clinically of a carcinoma will include dimpling or infiltration of the skin, deep fixation and a firm hard feel to the lump, which does not vary with the menstrual cycle. However, clinical diagnosis can be difficult and further investigation is usually indicated.

Examination of the breast area will delineate the position and extent of the tumour, its fixation and involvement of lymph nodes particularly in the axilla. Skin involvement is not uncommon with oedema of the skin giving the classical 'peau d'orange' appearance. Inflammation of the breast is seen with inflammatory carcinoma and is usually indicative of a very aggressive tumour. Other features of a locally advanced carcinoma are ulceration of the skin or skin nodules.

In some patients, particularly the elderly, the patient may present with an eczematous patchy rash over the nipple and surrounding areola. This condition, known as Paget's disease of the nipple, usually indicates intraduct carcinoma even in the absence of a palpable lump or mammographic abnormality.

Sometimes the presentation of breast cancer is with metastases, particularly to bone where both osteolytic and osteoblastic deposits may be found. Other presentations, such as pleural effusions, brain metastases and hypercalcaemia, are far less common.

Diagnosis

The diagnosis of breast cancer is based on a triple approach comprising clinical examination, mammography and aspiration cytology or biopsy.

If the diagnosis is confirmed, staging of the disease is important. There are several systems of staging but the TNM system is most useful. This can be simplified into a clinical staging (Table 8.2) or into three categories: operable breast cancer, locally advanced disease and metastatic disease.

A number of investigations should be performed at diagnosis including a haematological screen, biochemical profile and chest X-ray. For patients with large

Stage I	T1	N0	M0	
Stage IIA	T0	N1	M0	
	T1	N1	M0	
	T2	N0	M0	
Stage IIB	T2	N1	M0	Operable disease
	T3	N0	M0	
Stage IIIA	T0	N2	M0	
	T1	N2	M0	
	T2	N2	M0	
	T3	N1	M0	
Stage IIIB	T3	N2	M0	Inoperable
	T4	Any N	M0	locally advanced
	Any T	N3	M0	disease
Stage IV	Any T	Any N	M1	Metastatic disease

Abbreviations: T, tumour; N, node; M, metastasis.

Table 8.2 Clinical stage grouping based on TNM classification

tumours, locally advanced disease or features suggestive of metastases, additional investigations should be performed, including a radioisotopic bone scan. A liver ultrasound may also be indicated if liver function tests are abnormal.

Prognostic factors

As mentioned above, breast cancer can follow a variable clinical course. This can be predicted by a number of prognostic factors. These include tumour size, the presence of axillary lymph node metastases, histological type and grade, steroid receptor expression and various biological indices of cell proliferation and oncogene expression. Of all of these, axillary lymph node status is the most powerful prognostic factor with the prognosis deteriorating as the number of involved lymph nodes increases.

Management

Management of breast carcinoma is complex and provides many challenges. The three principal aims of treatment are:

- local control of the primary disease in the breast and regional lymph nodes
- prevention of metastases
- palliation of advanced metastatic disease.

Local control

Until the mid-1980s, mastectomy was the routine surgical treatment for carcinoma of the breast. However, loss of a breast is a mutilating surgical procedure which can create considerable psychological morbidity and problems with body image. Because of this, breast conserving surgery has developed, where the lump is removed by wide local excision and followed up by radiotherapy to the breast. Breast conserving surgery and radiotherapy is as good as mastectomy in achieving local control and does not prejudice the chances of long-term disease-free survival. The principal contraindications to this approach are multi-focal disease in the breast, a large tumour (over 4 cm) and extensive *in situ* carcinoma. Some patients still prefer mastectomy, even when technically this could be safely avoided. It is now generally accepted that the woman must be involved in decisions about her treatment.

Excision of the lump alone is an inadequate treatment, except possibly for very small well-differentiated tumours. With this exception, radiotherapy should be given to the whole breast and generally is followed by a boost dose to the scar area and tumour bed. Radiotherapy is given as an out-patient treatment on a daily basis (Monday to Friday), usually for 5–6 weeks.

Radiotherapy may also be indicated after mastectomy and is directed to the chest wall, anteriorly and laterally. Undoubtedly this reduces the chance of local recurrence but it may produce late toxicity such as cardiac damage and a risk of second malignancy. Because of this, if the breast cancer is small and excision margins well clear of the tumour, some specialists omit the routine use of post-operative radiotherapy.

The management of axillary lymph nodes remains an area of great debate. Surgical management of the axilla varies from none to a full clearance of the axillary contents with removal of lymph nodes at all three levels. Surgical clearance of the axilla reduces the chance of axillary recurrence to 1–2% and provides useful prognostic information on the number of lymph nodes involved. However, for some patients this extensive surgery is unnecessary and simply adds morbidity to the surgical management. Because of this, a sampling of lymph nodes is preferred by some surgeons to provide information on lymph node involvement in order to plan future treatment. In this situation, if the lymph nodes are found to be involved, radiotherapy is usually extended to include the axilla and supraclavicular lymph nodes.

The combination of radiotherapy and surgery to the axilla increases the probability of lymphoedema (brawny swelling of the arm) and certainly the combination of extensive axillary surgery and radical radiotherapy should be avoided. Radiotherapy to the internal mammary lymph nodes is now rarely performed.

Prevention of metastases

Since the mid-1980s, it has also become clear that drug treatment is very important to reduce the probability of developing metastatic disease. Systemic treatment reduces the chances of dying of breast cancer by about 30%, an effect which is maintained for at least 10 years. The type of drug treatment depends principally on the age of the patient. The older the patient, the more important endocrine treatment is, while chemotherapy is most clearly indicated in young patients. It is

Prognostic factors	Therapy
Pre-menopausal	
N+ve > 4 nodes	Doxorubicin × 4 → CMF × 6 → Tamoxifen
N+ve 1–3 nodes	CMF × 6 → Tamoxifen
N–ve + GIII or vascular invasion	CMF × 6 → Tamoxifen
N–ve + > 2 cm	Tamoxifen
N–ve + < 2 cm	None (under clinical trial)
Post-menopausal	
N+ve + < 5 years since menopause	CMF × 6 → Tamoxifen
N+ve + > 5 years since menopause	Tamoxifen
N–ve + > 2 cm	Tamoxifen
N–ve + < 2 cm	None

Abbreviations: CMF, cyclophosphamide, methotrexate, fluorouracil; G, histological grade; N, axillary lymph nodes.

Table 8.3 Adjuvant therapy policy for breast cancer based on prognostic factors

currently recommended that pre-menopausal women with lymph node involvement should receive six courses of combination chemotherapy while post-menopausal women should receive tamoxifen by mouth for at least 2 years. The value of adding endocrine therapy to chemotherapy in young women and conversely the addition of chemotherapy to endocrine treatment in older women remains an area of investigation. For women without involvement of the lymph nodes, recommendations for adjuvant therapy depend on other prognostic factors and the toxicity of the treatmentto be applied. Tamoxifen is more widely used because of its reduced side-effect profile compared with combination chemotherapy. Table 8.3 shows local policy in Sheffield based on these principles.

Advanced breast cancer

For the treatment of inoperable locally advanced disease, cytotoxic chemotherapy or hormonal therapy is appropriate in addition to radiotherapy. This is given with the aim of reducing the local tumour mass, healing ulceration and controlling bleeding or discharge. Combined modality treatments have led to modest improvements, mainly in local control of the disease, but chemotherapy has had little influence on the overall survival of these women. However, encouraged by the improvements seen following adjuvant chemotherapy in operable disease, there are currently several collaborative research groups testing the role of intensive chemotherapy in conjunction with bone marrow growth factors and bone marrow stem cell support in addition to radical surgery and/or radiotherapy to the breast.

For women with metastatic breast cancer, treatment is palliative. Nevertheless, unlike most other common cancers the clinical course can be long and 10–20% of women will be alive 5 years after the development of metastases. Endocrine therapy is the preferred initial treatment except in patients with rapidly deteriorating liver or lung function who should be considered for urgent chemotherapy. The efficacy of all endocrine treatments is similar but tamoxifen is the best tolerated and therefore the treatment of choice. Significant (over 50%) tumour shrinkage (a complete or partial objective response) following endocrine treatment occurs in one-third of unselected patients. It is more likely in those with either steroid receptor positive tumours, who have a long disease-free interval from diagnosis to relapse, and/or in those with bone or soft tissue metastases rather than visceral disease. Subsequent responses to different hormonal agents may occur but eventually the disease becomes endocrine resistant and chemotherapy is necessary if further control of the disease is to be achieved.

Chemotherapy will not be appropriate for all patients but, used appropriately, can produce very worthwhile palliation of symptoms without causing unacceptable toxicity. Furthermore, improvements in supportive care have improved the quality of life for patients requiring this treatment for advanced disease. Chemotherapy regimens will achieve objective response and symptomatic benefit in about one-half of patients treated. The precise choice of drugs and schedule of administration to obtain the best results is not yet certain and will vary from one patient or clinical problem to another. The anthracyclines, doxorubicin and epirubicin are particularly active but are too toxic for elderly or frail patients. Increased response rates are seen when combinations of drugs are administered at high dose, but there is no evidence to suggest that these regimens produce more durable responses and undoubtedly they are far more toxic. To maximize what is a fairly narrow cost–benefit advantage, attention to the control of side-effects and restriction to patients who have symptomatic or imminently symptomatic disease is recommended. By doing this, effective palliation and an improvement in the patient's quality of life is often possible.

The clinical course and pattern of metastases in breast cancer is very variable and treatment should take this into account. Liver metastases are often associated with a rapidly progressive, poorly differentiated tumour and, even with palliative chemotherapy, the prognosis is very poor. On the other hand, patients with bone metastases typically have more indolent disease, sometimes confined exclusively to the skeleton, which causes considerable morbidity including pain, fractures, hypercalcaemia and a steady decline in mobility and quality of life. In recent years, the bisphosphonates, which are specific inhibitors of osteoclast function, have been shown to reduce the rate of bone destruction (osteolysis) and skeletal-related morbidity.

For the immediate management of painful bone metastases, radiotherapy can be very effective. Recently it has been recognized that short courses of radiotherapy over 1–5 days are as effective as, and much more convenient than, conventional protracted fractionation regimens over 2–3 weeks.

For patients with cerebral metastases, steroids (usually dexamethasone) are recommended to control the headaches, nausea and vomiting and other symptoms of raised intracranial pressure. Cranial irradiation may also be helpful in maintaining palliation, particularly in those patients whose life is not immediately threatened by the presence of widespread visceral metastases.

Pleural effusions are seen commonly in advanced breast cancer, causing breathlessness and cough, and should be drained to provide symptomatic relief. For immediate management this is best done through a needle inserted under local anaesthetic into the pleural cavity, but to prevent recurrence of the effusion, tube drainage to dryness followed by instillation of a sclerosant agent such as tetracycline or bleomycin is recommended. Similarly, ascites should also be drained but in this situation, drugs injected into the peritoneal cavity are of little benefit.

Breast cancer in men

Breast cancer in men is uncommon, constituting no more than 1% of all cases of breast cancer. Associations are seen with Klinefelter's syndrome, and in men who have a family history of breast cancer in their female first-degree relatives. The pathology and clinical pattern are similar to that of breast cancer in women and the appropriate management by surgery, endocrine manipulation, radiotherapy and chemotherapy should also be along the lines given above for breast cancer in women.

9

Alimentary tract cancer

R E COLEMAN

The upper alimentary tract above the pharyngo-oesophageal junction is considered in Chapter 10; the remainder is discussed here under the headings: oesophagus; stomach; liver, pancreas and gall bladder; duodenum, jejunum and ileum; caecum, colon and rectum; anal canal and anus.

Oesophagus

Malignant tumours of the oesophagus represent about 5% of all cancers with 5000 new cases a year in the UK. They occur mainly in later life and are more common in men than in women. Smoking and alcohol consumption, particularly spirits, are the main aetiological factors. In addition, disorders of oesophageal motility or chronic acid reflux increase the risk of cancer.

The majority of oesophageal tumours are squamous cell carcinomas, arising in stratified epithelium. Adenocarcinomas account for about 15% of lesions and may arise at the lower end in gastric-type mucosa, which can extend a short distance up into the oesophagus. Tumours arise most often at one of the areas of partial natural narrowing of the oesophagus, namely the pharyngo-oesophageal junction (20%), the junction of upper and middle thirds where it is crossed by the left main bronchus (40%), and at the lower end where the oesophagus passes through the diaphragm (40%).

Local infiltration occurs early with both circumferential and longitudinal spread; the former results in stenosis, and by virtue of the latter the upper and lower limits of a tumour may extend well beyond those demonstrable by oesophagoscopy or radiology. Invasion of adjacent mediastinal structures may occur, particularly the trachea and main bronchi. Lymphatic spread also occurs early to mediastinal, neck and upper abdominal nodes, and is present in about 50% of tumours which are 5 cm or more in length. Distant metastatic spread is mainly to the liver through the portal venous system but also to the lungs and bones.

Symptoms and signs

The main symptom is slowly progressive dysphagia, initially for solids and later for fluids also. The level of the dysphagia can sometimes be fairly well localized by the patient. Any middle-aged or elderly patient with dysphagia should be investigated promptly and considered to have oesophageal cancer until proved otherwise. Retrosternal pain or discomfort and regurgitation may occur. Later, weight loss develops due to reduced calorie intake and the general effects of malignancy.

Investigations

The most valuable investigations are endoscopy (oesophagoscopy) and radiology (barium swallow). At oesophagoscopy a biopsy can be taken and the lumen dilated if necessary. CT of the chest and abdomen is useful to determine the extent of the lesion and detect lymph node and hepatic metastases before embarking on treatment with surgery or radiotherapy. Liver function tests and a chest X-ray should also be performed.

Management

Management depends on the level of the tumour, the degree of local spread, the presence of any metastases and the general condition of the patient. The upper third of the oesophagus is closely related to other vital structures in the mediastinum, and surgical clearance and reconstruction is often impossible. Middle third lesions are more accessible by the lateral transthoracic approach, and early tumours are resectable, although the operative mortality is 10–20%. Lower third tumours are the most accessible, by a combined thoracic and abdominal route. Excision is the only potentially curative treatment. The tumour is mobilized and resected with the proximal portion of the stomach followed by reanastomosis of the remaining oesophagus to the gastric remnant.

Radiotherapy is the treatment of choice for tumours of the upper oesophagus and radical high-dose treatment over 5–6 weeks is indicated for lesions up to 5 cm in length. During radiotherapy some temporary worsening of dysphagia is inevitable due to radiation oesophagitis, and nausea and vomiting are likely if the radiotherapy fields include the stomach or liver. Avoiding hot or cold foods, soothing medications, such as mucaine, anti-emetics and treatment of *Candida* super-infections will all reduce the toxicity of treatment. More extensive lesions which have infiltrated widely or produced lymph node metastases are beyond radical treatment. Palliative radiotherapy should be considered in these patients for relief of dysphagia; this is usually possible with short courses of radiotherapy with acceptable side-effects. Pre-operative and post-operative radiotherapy are advocated by some authorities, but do not appear to influence survival.

Palliation can also be achieved, sometimes with less upset, by endoscopy. Dilatation of a malignant stricture will partially relieve dysphagia and may be more effective if combined with insertion of a plastic tube to maintain a lumen (Atkinson or Celestin type). Endoprostheses are particularly useful in patients with recurrent aspiration of oesophageal contents into the lungs through a fistula. Alternatively, endoscopic laser coagulation of the tumour may relieve dysphagia and is helpful in controlling bleeding. Dietary advice, a liquidized diet and occasionally nasogastric or gastrostomy feeding may all help to improve the general strength and quality of life.

The results of treatment are disappointing, with overall survival figures of about 20% at 5 years for upper third tumours, 6% for middle third lesions, and 15% for those affecting the lower third.

Stomach

Gastric cancer is one of the most common malignancies of Western civilization; 12 000 new cases and 11 000 deaths occur each year in the UK. The highest incidence is in the sixth decade and the disease is twice as common in men as in women. Carcinogens from the diet and from the action of bacteria in the stomach are important in the development of the disease. Nitrosamines, tobacco, alcohol and smoked foods have all been implicated. Gastric cancer occurs three times more frequently in the absence of normal gastric secretion (achlorhydria). Chronic reflux of bile salts may also contribute and occurs freely following a gastrectomy or gastro-enterostomy. It is said that long-standing gastric ulcers can undergo malignant changes, but this has not been proved. Blood group O protects against gastric cancer while the incidence is increased in those with blood group A.

Most gastric cancers are adenocarcinomas; others include squamous carcinoma, lymphoma, leiomyosarcoma and carcinoid tumours, but the last two are very uncommon. Adenocarcinoma may be diffuse and infiltrating, fungating or ulcerated. The diffuse variety produces the classical 'leather bottle stomach' or linitis plastica. Local extension leads to invasion of adjacent structures. Lymphatic spread to local nodes occurs early. Later, deposits in the supraclavicular nodes, especially on the left in 'Virchow's node', become evident ('Troisier's sign'). Spread to the liver via the portal system is common. Transcoelomic spread also occurs and results in peritoneal disease often with ascites and deposits in the ovaries (Krukenberg tumours).

Symptoms and signs

Early symptoms are often vague. Appetite gradually deteriorates, and weight is slowly lost. Irregular mild upper abdominal discomfort or pain may be dismissed as 'indigestion'. Haematemesis or signs of pyloric obstruction may draw attention to the lesion. Anaemia is not uncommon. Later, an epigastric mass or hepatomegaly may be palpable and abdominal swelling due to ascites may develop.

Investigations

Investigations include a double-contrast barium meal examination, which may show an irregular filling defect or a rigid stomach wall, and gastroscopy, which also allows a biopsy to be taken. Distinction between a benign and malignant ulcer on barium meal may be difficult. A follow-up investigation is recommended with gast-roscopy if the lesion has not healed after 6 weeks of medical treatment. If surgery is contemplated, an ultrasound scan of the liver or abdominal CT is recommended to reduce the chances of operating on patients with inoperable or metastatic disease. Liver function tests and a chest X-ray should also be performed.

Treatment

The only radical treatment available is surgical excision of the stomach (gastrec-tomy) and adjacent lymph node groups. Only about 20% of patients have resectable disease and any chance of cure. A total gastrectomy is generally performed with careful dissection of the many regional lymph nodes. After the operation, the loss of stomach volume will lead to some feeding problems but usually the patient can adjust by taking small frequent meals. Vitamin B12 and sometimes iron supplements will be needed in those surviving more than a few months. Malabsorption and hypoglycaemia due to a 'dumping syndrome' may occur. Palliative surgery is often valuable in bypassing an obstructive lesion or to stop bleeding.

Radiotherapy has little to offer as a radical treatment owing to the dose-limiting toxicity which is inevitable in adjacent structures. Post-operative radiotherapy is of no proven value. Palliative radiotherapy which requires a lower dose is possible and may be helpful in relieving pain.

There is considerable interest in the role of chemotherapy, but its role is not defined. Adjuvant chemotherapy does not appear to improve survival. How-ever, there are encouraging reports that pre-operative chemotherapy will increase the proportion of patients who are able to undergo radical surgical resection. Palliation can sometimes be achieved with chemotherapy. Fluorouracil, particularly by infusion, anthracyclines, cisplatin and mitomycin C are the most useful agents. Responses occur in 30–50% of patients but are short lived and usually only achieved at a cost of considerable toxicity. Consequently, chemotherapy should only be given by specialist oncologists and within a clinical trial evaluating its usefulness.

Results

Only about 25% of patients who undergo radical surgery are alive after 5 years. Furthermore, many tumours are inoperable when diagnosed, with a median survival of 3–6 months. At present, the only real hope of improving results lies in earlier diagnosis when radical surgery is still possible.

Liver, pancreas and gall bladder

Malignant disease of these organs accounts for as many deaths as gastric cancer.

Liver

Primary malignancy of the liver (hepatoma) is one of the most common tumours worldwide but uncommon in the UK with 1100 new cases a year. The incidence is highest in oriental races, and four times higher in men than in women although this sex difference is less marked in Europe. In more than half the cases, it is associated with cirrhosis of the liver. The hepatitis B virus and mould toxins are known aetiological factors.

The tumour often arises from a cirrhotic nodule and may be multi-focal. The tumour cells are derived from hepatocytes and frequently stain with AFP, which can also be measured in the serum. The tumour invades the liver along the bile tracts, eventually penetrating the capsule and invading the adjacent structures. Peritoneal spread with ascites and lung metastases occur late.

Symptoms and signs

The main symptoms and signs are malaise, local pain due to stretching of the liver capsule and obstructive jaundice; haemorrhage into the tumour may cause severe pain. Later, a mass may be palpable, and swollen legs due to a combination of a low serum albumin and pressure on the inferior vena cava or signs of chronic liver disease may be present. In many cases, the level of serum AFP is raised, and this is a useful marker for diagnosis and the monitoring of response to treatment. The tumour may produce a variety of peptides which result in metabolic upset, such as hypercalcaemia, polycythaemia or hypoglycaemia.

Investigations

Extensive investigation is needed if surgical resection is contemplated. In addition to liver function tests, clotting studies, AFP and hepatitis antibodies, a CT scan of the chest and abdomen and hepatic angiography are necessary.

Treatment

Treatment is essentially surgical although results are poor, with less than 10% surviving after 5 years, as only 10–20% have operable disease. Partial hepatectomy, or in selected cases liver transplantation, provide the only chance of cure. Hepatic artery embolization is possible if the portal venous circulation is adequate for viability of the normal liver and provides temporary relief of pain. Chemotherapy is of limited value with occasional partial responses seen with anthracyclines and mitozantrone.

Pancreas

Adenocarcinoma of the pancreas is a disease of later life with 6000 new cases a year in the UK. It affects men slightly more frequently than women and is associated with smoking and pancreatitis. The tumour arises more often in the head of the organ than in the tail, but only in proportion to the amount of tissue in each part.

One-third of lesions are diffuse in origin; 90% of the tumours arise from the ducts and 10% from glandular elements and are almost invariably mucin-secreting adeno-carcinomas. Tumours of the insulin-producing islet cells are rare and completely different in histology and behaviour. The tumour infiltrates through the gland or spreads along the pancreatic duct to the ampulla of Vater where it may obstruct the flow of bile. Regional lymph node involvement and liver deposits occur early, and bone and lung metastases are not uncommon.

Signs and symptoms

Progress of the tumour is insidious. Jaundice, due to bile duct obstruction, is the cardinal sign of a lesion in the head of the pancreas, but usually indicates advanced disease. Back pain, which is typically constant and severe in nature, is a frequent symptom especially of tumours arising in the body or the tail. Malabsorption and steatorrhoea occasionally occur. Pancreatic cancer is associated with various dis-orders of coagulation including thrombophlebitis, disseminated intravascular coagulation (DIC), renal, splenic and portal vein thrombosis.

Investigations

Basic investigations include assessment of liver function, clotting studies, chest X-ray and an ultrasound or CT scan of the upper abdomen. Visualization of the pancreas is often difficult and this contributes to the typical delay in diagnosis. Histological confirmation is recommended and is usually possible by percutaneous CT-guided biopsy or endoscopy. Occasionally a laparotomy is necessary.

Treatment

Treatment is surgical; these tumours are resistant to radiotherapy and cytotoxic chemotherapy. Operability rates are low and 5-year survival figures are less than 1%. Palliative cholecystoduodenostomy for biliary drainage may be of temporary benefit. Pain relief may be difficult with standard analgesics and in such cases an anaesthetic or alcohol block to the coeliac plexus can be helpful. A biliary stent, inserted via an endoscope in the duodenum, provides useful relief of jaundice. Cholestyramine may be helpful for the pruritus of obstructive jaundice.

Gall bladder and bile ducts

Malignancy of the gall bladder and extrahepatic bile ducts is a disease of later life with 2300 cases a year in the UK. In contrast to primary liver cancer, it is almost four times as common in women as in men. Calculi are present in a high proportion of cases. The majority of lesions are adenocarcinomas, but about 10% are squam-ous cell carcinomas.

Symptoms

Symptoms are usually vague until a late stage of the disease when jaundice may occur. An exact diagnosis without laparotomy may be difficult. However, with modern endoscopic techniques of cannulating the common bile duct, detailed imaging of the biliary tract can be achieved which may identify the tumour and enable biopsy without resorting to a laparotomy.

Treatment

Radical treatment is often impossible because of local invasion, lymph node metastases, seedling deposits along the biliary tract, and distant metastases. Radiotherapy and cytotoxic chemotherapy are of no value. Palliative surgery to drain the biliary system, or insertion of a biliary stent either via an endoscope or following percutaneous cannulation of a bile duct in the liver is often the only treatment possible apart from sedatives and analgesics. With the exception of very early tumours discovered incidentally at cholecystectomy, 5-year survival figures are a mere 5–10%. The close association between gallstones and gall bladder cancer has been advanced as a strong argument in favour of cholecystectomy in all cases of gallstones.

Duodenum, jejunum and ileum

Malignant disease of these organs is rare. The only one warranting attention here is lymphoma, which occasionally arises in the Peyer's patches. Usually it is of non-Hodgkin's type. It presents as vague bowel upset, as obstruction or as a malabsorption syndrome. It is managed in the same way as lymphoma arising in other areas of lymphoid tissue, and the prognosis is similar with about 45% well at 5 years.

Small bowel carcinoid tumours are discussed in Chapter 19.

Caecum, colon and rectum

Cancer of the large bowel is common, and in white races accounts for more deaths than any other form of malignant disease. It occurs mainly in middle and old age, and affects men and women equally with 28 000 new cases a year in the UK. The principal sites are the caecum and ascending colon (15%), rectosigmoid region (40%) and rectum (35%).

Predisposing factors include single or multiple polyps, especially familial polyposis, and long-standing ulcerative colitis. It is now widely believed that carcinomas of the colon and rectum arise almost exclusively from pre-existing benign adenomas. Sluggish bowel movement has been incriminated, particularly in developed

Deletions or mutations

Adenomatous polyposis coli (APC) gene (chromosone 5)
Mutated in colon cancer (MCC) gene (chromosome 2)
c-Ki-RAS 2
P53 (chromosome 17)
Deleted in colon cancer (DCC) gene (chromosome 18)
Multiple allelic loss (altered allelotype)

Amplifications
c-MYC

Altered gene expression

Table 9.1   Genetic abnormalities in colorectal cancer

countries where the diet is low in residue and possibly high in carcinogens from food additives and preservatives. The genetics of colorectal cancer has been extensively researched recently and has identified multiple steps in the development of the cancer (Table 9.1).

Colorectal tumours are adenocarcinomas, sometimes with mucin production, and frequently stain for carcinoembryonic antigen. The tumour spreads circumferentially and longitudinally along the mucosa and invades through the bowel wall. Spread through the peritoneal cavity may result in ascites and lymph node and haematological spread are common, the latter principally through the portal circulation to the liver.

Symptoms and signs

Colorectal tumours may be of exophytic or ulcerative, infiltrative types. Blood and mucus in the faeces and a change in bowel habit with alternating constipation and diarrhoea are the most common presenting symptoms. The blood passed *per rectum* will be bright red if the tumour arises in the rectum or sigmoid and dark red and mixed in the stool if from the proximal colon. Anaemia may develop. Pain on defecation and a frequent urge to open the bowels are symptoms that patients may report in advanced rectal tumours. Later, evidence of subacute or acute intestinal obstruction supervenes. Around 20% of tumours present as a surgical emergency with obstruction or peritonitis due to perforation.

Rectal tumours may be palpable on digital rectal examination and about three-quarters of colorectal tumours arise within the range of a sigmoidoscope. Signs of metastatic disease, such as hepatomegaly or ascites, and rarely of fistulae to other organs, such as the bladder, may be evident.

Investigations

Investigations include sigmoidoscopy (or colonoscopy) and biopsy for accessible tumours and barium enema examination. The latter should be supplemented by air insufflation to obtain good quality double-contrast radiographs. Tumours and polyps larger than 1 cm can be visualized by barium enema. A chest X-ray and a liver ultrasound should be performed before elective surgery.

Conventionally, colorectal tumours are staged according to Dukes' classification: A, confined to the bowel wall; B, invasion through the bowel wall; C, involvement of regional lymph nodes; and D, presence of metastases. Most patients present with B and C lesions, 10% present with A tumours and 20% with D tumours.

Treatment

Surgery is the only curative treatment. Resection of the involved segment of the bowel with a wide margin to avoid leaving 'skip lesions' in the bowel and regional lymph nodes with end-to-end anastomosis is indicated. Tumours of the lower rectum may require abdominoperineal resection and a colostomy. However, modern surgical stapling suture techniques have reduced the amount of rectal tissue required to enable satisfactory anastomosis. Despite an 80% resection rate, almost half of patients will develop recurrent disease within 2 years, usually in the liver.

Palliative surgery is often required to bypass an obstructive lesion or create a defunctioning colostomy and provides good relief of symptoms. Recently, as surgery on the liver has become safer, resection of liver metastases is becoming more widely recommended. For patients with one to three lesions, especially if confined to one lobe of the liver, resection or partial hepatectomy is feasible and seems to improve prognosis with impressive results in the highly selected patients reported in the literature.

Radiotherapy is not relevant in the primary management of colonic tumours because of the radiosensitivity of normal neighbouring structures. However, radiotherapy is important in the management of rectal tumours. Pre-operative radiotherapy increases the proportion of rectal tumours which are resectable while post-operative radiotherapy significantly reduces local recurrence rates.

Until recently, chemotherapy has not appeared to be useful in colorectal cancer. However, important improvements in survival are now reported with adjuvant chemotherapy and useful palliation of advanced disease is possible with regimens which are well tolerated and acceptable to patients. Fluorouracil is the drug of choice in both situations. Response rates to fluorouracil alone given by bolus injection are low (5–20%) because of rapid metabolism. Many fluorouracil-containing combination chemotherapy regimens have been tried but have failed to improve significantly on these results and simply increased the toxicity of treatment. However, it is now understood that the efficacy of fluorouracil can be improved either by administering the agent over a long period of time to facilitate entry of drug into the cancer cells or by modulating its activity by the additional administration of folinic acid (see Chapter 5 for additional information). Treatment given in this way results in a 30–40% objective response rate and a 50–60% symptomatic rate of response.

In the adjuvant situation, fluorouracil-based chemotherapy reduces the probability of recurrence after apparently curative surgery by about one-third. Patients with Dukes' C tumours (lymph node positive) are increasingly being offered routine post-operative chemotherapy. Fluorouracil is given with either folinic acid or the immune stimulator levamisole for up to 1 year. Clinical trials continue, to investigate the best combination of drugs and duration of treatment.

Results

The prognosis of colorectal cancer depends on the Dukes' stage. The reported 5-year survival rates are 80% for Dukes' A, 60% for Dukes' B, 30% for Dukes' C and 5% for those with metastatic disease at presentation.

Anal canal and anus

Tumours of the anus are rare with about 300 cases a year in the UK. The mucosal lining of the anal canal differs from that of the rectum, being of cutaneous type. Therefore, the majority of cancers in this area are squamous cell carcinomas. The anus itself is covered by normal skin, and occasionally basal cell carcinomas are seen. Malignant melanomas occasionally arise in either area. Women are affected a little more frequently than men. Leucoplakia may undergo malignant change, and it has been suggested that haemorrhoids and fistulae predispose to carcinoma. Homosexual activity, specifically anal intercourse, is associated with the disease through sexual transmission of human papilloma viruses.

Most tumours are ulcerated and infiltrating. Lymphatic drainage is to the groin nodes, but deposits from extensive tumours may be found in the iliac and para-aortic lymph nodes. Distant metastases are rare at presentation.

Symptoms and signs

Early symptoms are local irritation and discomfort, tenesmus, discharge and bleeding. Pain is a late symptom. Tumours of the anal verge are visible on inspection and the others can be assessed by digital examination of the rectum and proctoscopy. Enlarged inguinal nodes may be palpable.

Investigation

Biopsy, either directly or via a proctoscope, should be performed along with fine needle cytology of palpable lymph nodes. In some cases, examination under anaesthetic will be required. A CT scan of the pelvis is helpful in assessing deep invasion of the tumour and the presence of pelvic lymph nodes in advanced lesions. Liver ultrasound and chest X-ray should be performed as a screen for metastases.

Treatment

Anal margin tumours can be treated by wide local excision. For anal canal tumours there is a move away from abdominoperineal resection to radical radiotherapy with or without chemotherapy. Radiotherapy allows sphincter preservation and avoids the effects of surgery on bladder and sexual function. Treatment is given initially to the pelvis and inguinal lymph nodes with a boost by either external beam therapy or a radioactive implant. The local radiation reaction is very uncomfortable for the patient but subsides a few weeks after completing treatment.

Chemotherapy with fluorouracil and mitomycin C given in combination with radiotherapy appears to improve the results of radiotherapy with a higher complete response rate and fewer cases requiring surgical salvage.

Results

The overall 5-year survival is about 70%, with small early lesions and those at the anal verge doing best.

10

Head and neck cancer

M H ROBINSON

Head and neck cancers represent less than 1.5% of patients referred to standard oncology centres. However, the complexity of their management results in a disproportionately high workload. Squamous carcinoma in the head and neck in the UK is primarily due to smoking. A high consumption of alcohol significantly increases the risk from smoking. A number of industrial diseases are associated with head and neck cancer, including adenocarcinomas acquired from working with hard wood. These tumours usually arise in the nasal cavity or sinuses. In the Indian subcontinent the chewing of tobacco and betel nut leaves is associated with oral cavity tumours. In South-East Asia, EBV is an aetiological factor in the development of nasopharyngeal carcinoma.

The head and neck is a complex area with many different structures (Table 10.1).

Most (90%) of the tumours occurring on the upper area of the digestive tract are epithelial and of squamous type. Adenocarcinomas occur in less than 5% of cases particularly in the salivary glands and thyroid. Other tumours (e.g. sarcomas and melanomas) occur less commonly.

Spread of cancer

Squamous carcinomas may be either exophytic, ulcerative or infiltrative in type. Their local aggressiveness may be associated with their differentiation, which varies from undifferentiated to well differentiated. Tumours of the floor of the mouth may become very large before symptoms drive the patient to the GP. Tumours of the nasopharynx, although not large, may involve a number of sensitive structures before presentation. This can result in cranial nerve lesions for example, 3, 4, 6. At other tumour sites, symptoms occur early in the natural history. Patients may notice hoarseness when tumours of the vocal cords are less than 1 cm in size.

Involvement of lymph nodes is very common following development of a squamous cell carcinoma in the head and neck. The incidence of lymph node involvement varies according to site. Of patients with nasopharyngeal carcinoma 80–90% present with involved lymph nodes compared with less than 15% of patients with maxillary antral tumours. Other sites commonly associated with lymph node metastases are the oropharynx and hypopharynx. The lymph nodes draining the head and neck are in the pre-auricular, submental, submandibular

- Lip
- Mouth
    - Tongue
    - Floor of mouth
    - Buccal and gingival mucosa
    - Palate
    - Mandible and maxilla
- Oropharynx
    - Tonsil
    - Posterior third of tongue
    - Retromolar trigone
- Postnasal space
- Nasal cavity and paranasal sinuses
- Laryngopharynx
    - Larynx
    - Hypopharynx
    - Upper oesophagus
- Ear
- Salivary glands
- Thyroid and parathyroids
- Eyelids

Table 10.1   Structures in the head and neck area

and deep cervical areas. Overall, the most common site for lymph node metastases is in the upper deep cervical (jugulo-digastric) nodes.

Treatment

Curative treatment for head and neck cancer involves the choice of surgery, radiotherapy or a combination. There is no proven role for adjuvant chemotherapy in the treatment of squamous carcinoma of the head and neck.

Squamous carcinomas are relatively radiosensitive compared with adenocarcinomas, sarcomas and melanomas. Surgery and radiotherapy are equally effective in eliminating small volume squamous carcinomas in most sites of the head and neck. The choice between surgery and radiotherapy should be determined following preliminary discussions between the surgeon and oncologist. Radiotherapy is usually the first choice, where surgery would be associated with significant functional loss. With increasing tumour stage there is an increasing role for surgery and in most advanced tumours (usually those greater than 4 cm) a combination of surgery and radiotherapy may be indicated. Radiotherapy is also extremely effective in eliminating microscopic residual disease left by the surgeon at the margins of the excision. Extremely advanced tumours may be palliated by radiotherapy, chemotherapy or occasionally surgical intervention.

The advantages of surgery to the patient are that it is quicker and that the lesion is seen to be removed and the patient may leave hospital within 2 weeks.

Radiotherapy is delivered over a period of 3–6.5 weeks depending on the size of the tumour and the training of the oncologist. Side-effects from radiotherapy to the head and neck can be quite severe. Mucositis develops 2–3 weeks into the course of treatment and this may severely impair the patient's ability to gain adequate nutrition. Nasogastric or gastrostomy feeding may be necessary. Acute reactions from radiotherapy may settle down within a month of its completion and late problems are unusual. Small oral primary tumours may be treated by interstitial radiotherapy using an iridium-192 implant. This has the advantage of delivering a high local dose while minimizing the dose to other normal tissues. Such an implant is left *in situ* for 6–7 days. In thyroid cancer, oral administration of ^{131}I is used for well-differentiated follicular tumours. This is preferentially taken up by the thyroid following initial surgery and may be used to treat metastatic disease.

Lymph node metastases

Conventionally, lymph node involvement is treated by surgery. However, lymph nodes of less than 2 cm in size associated with a small radio-curable primary can be treated by radiotherapy. Outside this situation, radical neck dissection is indicated for overtly involved unilateral lymph node disease. This involves the removal *en bloc* of the sternomastoid muscle, internal jugular vein, upper middle and lower deep cervical, submandibular and submental lymph nodes and submandibular salivary gland, nodes in the supraclavicular fossa and posterior triangle of the neck, with all the intervening lymphatic channels and connective tissue. In certain circumstances this operation may be modified to a functional neck dissection with less morbidity. Where the risk of occult lymphatic involvement is greater than 30% elective nodal radiation is of value in reducing this risk. This is particularly useful where patients are unlikely to attend for careful routine follow-up.

Lip

This is the most common site of malignant tumours in the mouth area accounting for about 25%. Tumours of the lower lip are about 10 times more common than those of the upper lip. They usually occur in elderly patients. They usually present early and may be cured by radiotherapy or surgery. The choice depends on the potential functional or cosmetic result. Predisposing factors include leucoplakia and prolonged exposure to sunlight.

Mouth

Tongue

Histologically, tumours of the tongue are almost all squamous carcinomas mainly of well-differentiated type. Adenocarcinomas occasionally arise from mucous glands of salivary tissue. Melanomas rarely occur. Tumours of the posterior third of the tongue tend to be less differentiated; lymphomas, predominantly of non-Hodgkin's type, are occasionally seen.

The tongue is the second most common site of malignant tumours in the mouth area (about 20%). Men are affected much more often than women. Aetiological factors include chronic irritation, as from a sharp tooth, habitual tongue biting and leucoplakia. About three-quarters of tumours arise on the anterior two-thirds of the tongue, the most common sites being the lateral border, dorsum, tip and under surface, in decreasing order of frequency. Macroscopically, lesions may be solid and nodular, softer and papillary, flat and plaque like, ulcerated and indurated or fissured.

Symptoms of early disease are absent or negligible. Local pain and ulceration may develop later. Reduced mobility of the tongue with dysphagia is usually a late feature. There may be excessive salivation. Lesions of the posterior third may present as a persistent sore throat. At presentation, lymph node involvement is evident in about one-third of anterior lesions and in about two-thirds of posterior lesions.

Tumours, less than 3 cm in size, occurring in the oral cavity may be cured by interstitial implant or surgery. Larger tumours may require external beam radiotherapy or more extensive surgery. Treatment of posterior-third lesions is predominantly by radiotherapy; the only surgical treatment is total glossectomy with severe functional consequences.

The local control rates for small anterior two-third tongue lesions are in excess of 90%. Overall 5-year survival is approximately 70%. The success rate drops rapidly with increasing stage.

Results of treatment of posterior-third tongue lesions are not as good. The overall 5-year survival varies between 60% and 25% depending on the stage. Approximately two-thirds of patients with posterior-third tongue lesions have lymph node involvement on presentation.

Floor of mouth

Tumours on the floor of the mouth account for some 15% of malignant mouth tumours. They are almost invariably squamous carcinomas. Early lesions away from the mandible may be treated by interstitial implantation. However, they commonly extend to or involve the mandible, in which case surgery is most commonly used. This may involve resection of the mandible and reconstruction using bone implants. As in other sites, node-negative patients do well with survival reduced by half where neck node involvement occurs.

Buccal and gingival mucosa tumours

In the Indian sub-continent, South-East Asia and the Philippines, the sucking of betel nut, tobacco and slaked lime plugs is often the cause of these types of tumour. In the UK this is rarely the case. However, leucoplakia as a predisposing factor is common. The principles of treatment are as described above for other sites. Early lesions may be treated by interstitial therapy. More advanced lesions are treated with external beam radiotherapy; surgery has a limited place.

Palate

Palatal tumours are rare. On the hard palate, tumours of salivary tissue are predominant. Adenoid cystic carcinomas are not uncommon. These have a considerable potential for local recurrence and a tendency to spread along nerves and to metastasize to the lung. Treatment of these lesions is primarily surgical with post-operative radiotherapy.

Tumours of the soft palate are predominantly squamous carcinomas and usually treated by radiotherapy.

Mandible and maxilla

Tumours of mandible and maxilla include sarcomas and adamantinomas. The latter is extremely rare, affecting women more than men; it is most common in the mandible. It arises from epithelial remnants in the bone. Rarely, malignant forms are described. Treatment of bony tumours is primarily surgical.

Tonsil and retromolar trigone

Tumours of the tonsillar fossa are commonly squamous carcinomas. However, lymphomas and lymphoepitheliomas also occur in this site. Early stage carcinomas of the tonsillar region can be treated successfully by external beam radiotherapy. This can be directed to cover the ipsilateral tonsil and first station lymph nodes alone. More advanced lesions are probably best treated by a combination of surgery and radiotherapy. The results of treatment of early cancer are good with 70–90% local control at 5 years. Although the principles of treatment for retromolar trigone lesions are the same as for tonsillar tumours the results are more disappointing.

Postnasal space

This is a small cavity but is centrally placed and tumours arising from its walls can have marked effects. In the UK, the instances are very low, but in China and South-East Asia it is much higher. In these countries it is associated with infection with EBV.

The most common type of tumours are squamous cell carcinomas, usually poorly differentiated and sometimes showing lymphocytic infiltration (lymphoepithelioma). Transitional cell carcinomas are described, and occasionally lymphomas arise in this area. Chordoma, a tumour of notocord remnants, may present in the postnasal space. Plasmacytomas and tumours of salivary gland tissue are also described.

Increasing local tumour bulk may cause nasal obstruction, discharge and bleeding, and occlusion of the Eustachian tube with deafness. The soft palate may be displaced downwards. Infiltration in the lateral and posterior walls is directed upwards by the dense pharyngeal fascia, with invasion of the foramina in the base of the skull and involvement of the bone itself cranial nerve palsies result (3rd,

4th, 5th and 6th at the foramen lacerum and 9th, 10th, 11th and 12th in the region of the foramen ovale). The tumour may extend into the orbit and produce proptosis.

Lymph node involvement is present in 80–90% at presentation and is commonly bilateral. MRI and CT scans are invaluable in determining the extent of the disease.

Results of treatment are unsatisfactory with an overall 5-year survival of 25%. However, radiotherapy is usually employed. A large volume of mucosa is treated including all mucosa. The areas at risk of spread include the back of the orbit, the nasal cavity and the base of the skull to the mediastinum.

Nasal cavity and paranasal sinuses

These must be considered as a whole, as the intercommunications between the nasal cavity and the sinuses often lead to extensive involvement of both by malignant tumours.

Tumour types include squamous cell carcinoma (about 80%), malignant salivary tumours, malignant melanoma, lymphoma and sarcoma. There may be a long history of chronic nasal catarrh and polyposis. The most common site of origin is the maxillary sinus (antrum). It is a small cavity and symptoms and signs are usually related to extension through the antral walls. Medial extension produces nasal obstruction, discharge and bleeding. Extension anteriorly leads to swelling of the cheek, initially in the malar areas, often with local pain and discomfort. Posterior extensions into the pterygoid fossa produce trismus. Upward extension through the thin bony floor of the orbit leads to diplopia and proptosis, and may result in numbness of the cheek due to the involvement of the maxillary division of the trigeminal nerve. Extension downwards produces swelling of the palate, alveolus or bucco-alveolar sulcus, and antral tumours may present initially in this area.

In the nasal cavity, common sites of origin are the septum and turbinates (especially the inferior). The ethmoid air cells are seldom involved alone, but are often affected in association with antral tumours. The classical sign is swelling in the inner canthus of the eye. Frontal sinus tumours are very uncommon, and sphenoidal sinus tumours are rare.

Treatment is by irradiation, or a combination of radiation and surgery. Overall results show 30% survival after 5 years.

Larynx and hypopharynx

Larynx

Malignant tumours of the larynx are the most common head and neck cancers other than skin tumours. Men are affected nine times more frequently than women, and almost all tumours are squamous cell carcinomas. The majority of laryngeal carcinomas arise in the glottic area, on the true cords, usually starting in the anterior third and spreading directly to the anterior commissure and opposite cord, to the arytenoid region and to the ventricle and subglottic area. Lateral extension results in reduced morbidity of the cord.

There are few lymphatic vessels in the true cord, and the lymph node deposits from early tumours are uncommon. However, once a tumour has spread beyond the cord it reaches tissue well supplied with lymphatics and node deposits are common. Supraglottic tumours produce node deposits early in their history. Subglottic tumours are rare and may develop nodes around the trachea and down into the mediastinum rather than the neck.

Hoarseness is the only early symptom of glottic carcinoma, and hoarseness persisting for more than 4 weeks should be regarded with suspicion. It may be intermittent initially but later becomes continuous. Later symptoms include local pain and dysphagia, irritant cough and dyspnoea.

Fibreoptic laryngoscopy is invaluable in making a diagnosis and staging these tumours. Direct laryngoscopy is mandatory, as are biopsies. CT is useful to determine the extension to the ventricle or subglottic region.

Tumours of the glottis are usually treated with radiotherapy in Europe. Between 66% and 90% of such lesions are cured by radiotherapy alone. About 50% of larger lesions may be considered curable with half the remainder being salvaged by laryngectomy. Laryngectomy is indicated for transglottic or bulky tumours. Incurable advanced disease may be treated by palliative radiotherapy. Early supraglottic lesions confined to one site, in a patient with a good airway, may be treated with radical radiotherapy. They are otherwise treated by laryngectomy.

Hypopharynx and upper oesophagus

The results of treatment of the hypopharynx are dismal. The two common sites for these tumours are the pyriform fossa and the postcricoid area. Lymph-node metastases develop early, and may be evident before any symptoms referrable to the primary tumour have been detected.

Pyriform fossa tumours are associated with discomfort in the throat, dysphagia and hoarseness. Lateral extension may make the primary mass palpable externally. Pain referred to the ear is not uncommon. The primary tumour is often difficult to visualize on indirect laryngoscopy. The most effective treatment is probably radical surgery by laryngopharyngectomy. The medical condition of many patients precludes this. Postcricoid tumours are associated with iron deficiency anaemia and the Plummer–Vinson syndrome. Dysphagia is the most common symptom and lymph node deposits are common. The principles of the treatment of this and the upper oesophagus are similar to that for pyriform fossa tumours.

Ear

The majority of tumours of the pinna, external auditory canal and middle ear are squamous carcinomas. The general principles of treatment described above apply.

Salivary glands

Tumours of the parotid, submandibular, and sublingual glands account for 3–4% of all neoplasms of the head and neck. The average age for malignant tumours is 55 years and for benign tumours about 40 years. About one-quarter of parotid tumours and one-half of submandibular tumours are malignant. About 80% of the major salivary gland tumours occur in the parotid.

Benign mixed tumours

These are the most common neoplasms of the salivary glands first appearing in patients in their early 20s. They are discrete slow growing tumours surrounded by an imperfect pseudocapsule. The primary treatment of these lesions is adequate surgery. Some tumours recur many times and display locally aggressive behaviour despite a benign histology.

Malignant tumours

These may be low or high grade in type. Surgical resection is usually adequate treatment for low-grade lesions whereas radiotherapy may be required as an adjuvant for high-grade lesions.

Thyroid and parathyroids

Thyroid carcinoma is a relatively rare disease representing a spectrum of cancers with different clinical behaviours. The disease occurs primarily in young and middle-aged adults. The peak incidence of papillary carcinoma occurs 15–20 years earlier than that of follicular carcinoma which is about 10 years before anaplastic carcinoma. Metastases are usually lymphatic from papillary carcinoma and haematogenous (bone, lung) from follicular carcinoma.

Most medullary carcinomas (approximately 80%) occur sporadically. However, they may also occur as part of multiple endocrine neoplasia types IIA and IIB. Type IIA is inherited as an autosomal dominant and type IIB is sporadic.

The treatment for thyroid cancer is predominantly surgical. Suppression of thyroid stimulating hormone (TSH) by exogenous thyroxine following ablation of residual thyroid activity with ^{131}I is valuable in papillary and follicular carcinomas. Metastatic tumour may also be treated with ^{131}I. Endocrine treatment is not of value in medullary or anaplastic carcinoma.

Parathyroid cancer is very rare. Less than 5% of all parathyroid tumours are malignant, usually with an indolent natural history after surgery.

Eyelids

Tumours of the eyelids are usually basal cell carcinomas. These may be treated by either local excision or radiotherapy. Where surgery may lead to exposure of the cornea, radiotherapy is used. With appropriate shielding the functional results are excellent.

Summary

The treatment of head and neck cancer represents a major challenge. It is crucial to employ a multidisciplinary team including surgeon, oncologist, dietitian, nurse specialist and speech therapist. The results of treating early lesions may be excellent, but in a number of sites the late presentation of patients is associated with dismal results. It is vital that the treatment of these tumours is centralized so that the appropriate level of expertise may be gained.

11

Cancer of the female genital tract

R E COLEMAN

Uterine cervix

Worldwide, carcinoma of the cervix is the third most common malignancy in women with about 4500 cases each year in the UK. It predominantly affects women in their 40s and 50s but is showing an increase in younger age groups. The highest levels are found in South America where the incidence reaches 100 in 100 000 compared with 12 in 100 000 in the UK.

Aetiology

The disease is more common in lower socio-economic groups. The age of first intercourse and of first pregnancy are important aetiological factors. The disease is more common in women who have had multiple partners. Viral infection with both herpes simplex type II and human papilloma virus type 16 and 18 have been implicated in the aetiology. Evidence for a viral cause is supported by the identification of high-risk men who have more than one partner who subsequently develops cervical cancer.

Screening

Invasive squamous carcinoma is generally preceded by *in situ* malignant change for 10 years or more. Because of this, routine cervical smear examination has been introduced in the UK to screen for the disease. Although only about one-third of cases with *in situ* change progress to malignancy, cervical screening can detect those at high risk so that treatment or close follow-up can be instituted. Dysplastic and *in situ* change are generally treated by either colposcopy or cone biopsy of the cervix.

Routine cervical smear testing has been associated with a marked decline in the incidence and severity of invasive cervical carcinoma. In the UK, the incidence has fallen by about 30%. It is recommended that all sexually active women below the age of 50 years have a cervical smear performed at 3–5 year intervals. Unfortunately women at particularly high risk often have the poorest compliance with screening programmes.

Pathology

About 90% of cancers are squamous cell in origin, arising from the epithelium of the vaginal cervix or endocervical canal. The rest are usually adenocarcinomas arising from the endocervix. Rarely sarcomas, particularly mixed mesodermal tumours, lymphoma, leukaemia and small cell carcinoma occur.

Invasive tumours may be exophytic or infiltrating and ulcerative. Typically, a proliferative growth on the cervix with surface ulceration is seen but occasionally a diffuse infiltrating tumour with intact mucosa due to tumour arising in the cervical canal develops. Locally the disease spreads to the vaginal fornices, the upper vaginal wall and body of the uterus.

Lymphatic spread occurs early with lymph node involvement found in 15% of stage I tumours. Initially lymphatic spread is to the paracervical nodes and from there to internal and external iliac, pre-sacral and obturator nodes and then on up to the para-aortic lymph node chain. The disease may spread along the broad and utero-sacral ligaments to involve the pelvic side wall or in severe cases infiltrate in to the bladder or rectum. Blood-borne metastases are less common but do occur, particularly to the bones and lungs. In many cases, however, the disease remains confined to the pelvis until very advanced.

Symptoms and signs

Early cervical carcinoma is asymptomatic, with the diagnosis typically made following an abnormal cervical smear. Later, bleeding and discharge are features occurring particularly after intercourse. The discharge is often blood-stained and offensive. Advanced disease may cause pain due to infiltration of pelvic nerves and ultimately may lead to a vesico-vaginal or recto-vaginal fistula and/or a ureteric obstruction.

Para-aortic lymphadenopathy may cause low back pain and patients with metastatic disease may have general symptoms of malignancy including malaise and weight loss.

Pelvic examination is essential to identify the tumour and assess extension into the vaginal mucosa and any evidence of spread into the parametrium or rectal mucosa. Routine investigations should include a full blood count, serum, urea and electrolytes and a chest X-ray. Examination under anaesthetic, including cystoscopy, should always be performed, at which time biopsies can also be taken. Usually a CT scan of the abdomen and pelvis is performed to assess local extension and enlargement of pelvic and para-aortic lymph nodes. Intravenous pyelography may be helpful to identify ureteric obstruction. Lymphangiography is now rarely required as most enlarged lymph nodes can be clearly seen on CT.

Staging of disease

Clinical staging is an essential preliminary to determining management. The FIGO staging system is generally accepted and is shown in Table 11.1.

Stage I
a Micro-invasive disease limited to the cervix
b Confined to the cervix with invasion of >5 mm

Stage II
a Extension into the upper two-thirds of the vagina
b Extension to the parametrium but not reaching the pelvic side wall

Stage III
a Extension to the lower third of the vagina
b Extension to the pelvic side wall

Stage IV
a Involvement of bladder or rectal mucosa
b Distant metastases

Table 11.1   FIGO staging for cancer of the cervix

Treatment

Radical treatment should be considered for all patients except those with stage IV disease. Occasionally, patients will present in renal failure due to bilateral ureteric obstruction. In selected cases, insertion of nephrostomy tubes to relieve renal obstruction may be performed prior to radical treatment with reasonable long-term results.

Disease confined to the cervix (stage I)

Radical radiotherapy and surgery are effective treatments in this situation. Radical surgery is usually the treatment of choice in young fit patients. A radical hysterectomy (Wertheim's) is performed during which, in addition to the removal of the uterus, fallopian tubes and ovaries, the upper vagina, parametrium and pelvic lymph nodes are also included in the resection.

Post-operative radiotherapy is indicated when there is involvement of removed pelvic lymph nodes or if the excision margins are not well clear of the tumour.

The results of radical radiotherapy for stage I cervical carcinoma are similar to those achieved by surgery. However, there may be more long-term morbidity following damage to the bladder and bowel. Because of this, radical radiotherapy is usually reserved for elderly patients, those medically unfit for surgery, or those who refuse surgery.

Radical radiotherapy usually involves external beam treatment to a dose of 40–50 Gy over 4–5 weeks plus intracavitary treatment to the cervix using an intra-uterine tube and vaginal source to give a further 25–30 Gy to the cervix and surrounding tissues.

Radical radiotherapy often produces temporary bowel dysfunction with pain on defecation and diarrhoea due to reaction in the rectal mucosa. Frequency and dysuria from reaction in the bladder base occurs towards the end of the treatment and for a week or two thereafter. Severe radiation changes in the rectum, bladder and bowel may lead to stricture formation in the rectum or sigmoid colon and occasional fistula formation. In addition, shortening and fibrosis of the vagina occurs, often resulting in problems with sexual activity. This can be miminized with good counselling of patients plus the provision of vaginal dilators, oestrogen replacement and lubricants.

Following radical treatment, particularly in young women, hormone replacement therapy should always be considered and is quite safe.

Tumours extended beyond the cervix (stages II and III)

In this situation, radical radiotherapy is usually the treatment of choice. The whole pelvis is treated by external beam therapy as above. Studies are in progress assessing the value of adding chemotherapy to radical radiotherapy. At present there is no indication for the routine use of chemotherapy and this treatment approach should still be considered experimental.

Extensive pelvic disease or metastases (stage IV)

In this situation, treatment should be considered palliative. Palliative radiotherapy for locally advanced disease may be helpful, particularly to control bleeding and pain. Palliative surgery in the form of a colostomy may be required when there is a recto-vaginal fistula. Chemotherapy for advanced disease has been quite extensively tested in recent years. Relief of symptoms and objective remissions are seen with drug schedules including cisplatin, methotrexate and ifosfamide. There is no evidence that combination therapy is superior to single agent treatment and all of these drugs have considerable associated toxicity.

Invasive cervical carcinoma diagnosed during pregnancy may be difficult to manage. If the fetus has reached viability (30 weeks), caesarean section is undertaken, and external radiation therapy is started as soon as the skin sutures have been removed. Intracavitary radioisotope therapy is given after external beam treatment, as by this time, involution of the uterus will be almost complete. If the pregnancy is less than 24 weeks, therapeutic abortion is to be recommended with radiotherapy immediately thereafter. Patients presenting in the intervening period require individual assessment.

Prognosis

The results of treatment are very much related to the stage at presentation. The 5-year survival rates are approximately 80% for stage I tumours (although those with Ib tumours and involved lymph nodes do considerably worse than this); 65% for stage II; 20–30% for stage III and less than 5% for stage IV.

Endometrium

This disease generally affects an older, predominantly post-menopausal, group of women. The incidence in the UK is similar to that of cervical cancer with about 4000 cases a year.

In contrast to cervical carcinoma, it is common in the nulliparous and those of low parity. It is also more common in obese women and those with diabetes. Endometrial carcinoma is related to prolonged oestrogen stimulation. Unopposed oestrogens, used as hormone replacement therapy, increase the incidence of endometrial carcinoma but this can be avoided by combined preparations incorporating progesterone and continuation of monthly menstruation following oestrogen withdrawal. Endometrial carcinoma is a recognized complication of oestrogen-secreting tumours of the ovary. In addition, there has been considerable publicity surrounding the slightly increased incidence of endometrial carcinoma following prolonged use of tamoxifen for breast cancer.

Pathology

Most endometrial cancers are adenocarcinomas, sometimes showing areas of squamous metaplasia. Rarely carcinosarcomas and mixed mesodermal tumours are reported. Pre-cancerous conditions include endometrial hyperplasia and polyps. The disease tends to remain localized within the pelvis with slow invasion of the myometrium followed by spread to the cervix and vaginal walls and deposits in the ovaries. Lymph node deposits and blood-borne metastases arise late. When metastases do occur they most frequently involve the lungs and bone.

Symptoms and signs

Endometrial carcinoma typically presents as post-menopausal bleeding. This may be heavy with the presence of clots. Occasionally in pre-menopausal women, irregular or intra-menstrual bleeding is seen. Vaginal discharge is less common. There may be a sense of discomfort in the pelvis but more general symptoms of malignancy, if present, are usually mild.

Pelvic examination may reveal a bulky uterus and vaginal discharge or bleeding from the cervical os may be visible.

Investigations

The diagnosis depends on histological examination of the uterine curettings. Other causes of abnormal menstrual bleeding need to be considered, including atrophic vaginitis and fibroids. Routine investigations should include a full blood count because chronic blood loss is common. Uterine curettage can now often be performed in the out-patient clinic, but occasionally examination under anaesthetic and dilatation of the cervical canal is necessary to allow formal uterine curettage to be

Stage I
a Confined to the endometrium and no myometrial invasion
b Confined to the endometrium with <50% myometrial invasion
c Confined to the endometrium but with >50% invasion

Stage II
Invasion of the cervix

Stage III
Spread into surrounding pelvic tissue

Stage IV
a Involvement of the bladder or rectum
b Distant metastases

Table 11.2 FIGO staging for cancer of the endometrium

performed. A chest radiograph is generally performed to exclude distant metastases. A CT scan is preferable to lymphangiography to assess local spread and lymph node status.

Staging

Carcinoma of the endometrium is also staged using the FIGO system as shown in Table 11.2.

Treatment

The disease is generally managed surgically with total abdominal hysterectomy and bilateral salpingectomy for disease localized to the endometrium and the more extensive Wertheim's hysterectomy if the cervix is also involved. If patients are unfit for surgery, radical external beam radiotherapy plus intracavitary treatment can be effective.

Post-operative radiotherapy is recommended for patients with poorly differentiated tumours and those with significant invasion of the myometrium or lymph node involvement.

Patients with locally advanced tumours and/or metastases may respond to progestogens; either medoxyprogesterone acetate or megestrol acetate can be used. The objective response rate is around 25% with more patients experiencing subjective benerit. There are no data to recommend routine prescription of adjuvant hormone therapy after local treatment. Chemotherapy is generally unhelpful for palliation.

Prognosis

The prognosis for endometrial carcinoma is generally good with 85% 5-year survival for stage I disease.

Ovary

Ovarian cancer affects 5000 women in the UK and causes 4000 deaths each year. The disease tends to occur in women over the age of 40 years and is more common in the nulliparous and in those from higher socio-economic groups. A familial pattern is seen in some cases, particularly in those occurring at an early age, and there is a recognized association with breast carcinoma. One of the genes responsible for susceptibility to ovarian cancer has been identified on chromosome 17 making molecular screening a possibility for the future.

Screening

Because ovarian cancer presents so late, attempts have been made to screen the disease using serum CA 125 measurements and abdominal or transvaginal ultrasound. Unfortunately, apart from in those with a strong family history, routine screening cannot be justified.

Pathology

Most ovarian tumours are of epithelial origin. The tumours typically have a mixture of solid and cystic components with the latter containing either serous or mucinous material. Serous cystadenocarcinomas typically show a papillary pattern. Other epithelial tumours include those with endometrioid differentiation and clear cell carcinomas.

The non-epithelial ovarian tumours are found in fewer than 5% of cases but include those derived from gonadal stroma, such as the granulosa cell and Sertoli cell tumours, which may produce oestrogens or androgens, respectively, and germ cell tumours. Dysgerminoma is the counterpart of the seminoma of the testis and is similarly very radiosensitive and chemosensitive. Benign teratoma (dermoid) is relatively common whereas malignant teratoma of the ovary is extremely rare. However, when it does occur it is managed in the same way as testicular teratoma.

Malignant ovarian tumours spread primarily by local extension and peritoneal seeding. Lymphatic spread to the para-aortic, mediastinal and supraclavicular lymph nodes occurs and haematogenous spread may result in lung and liver metastases. Pleural effusions are quite common. These may either have the features of a transudate and be cytologically negative for carcinoma cells (Meig's syndrome), or be frankly malignant, in which case they indicate a poor prognosis.

Symptoms and signs

Ovarian cancer often remains asymptomatic for some time and usually presents with vague symptoms of abdominal discomfort and pelvic pain due to solid or cystic tumour, ascites or both. Urinary frequency or incontinence and diarrhoea or constipation result from local pressure effects. Vague backache is not uncommon but severe pain is seldom present. Lower limb oedema may develop. Abnormal vaginal bleeding occurs, especially with oestrogen-secreting tumours.

Clinically, abdominal swelling and distension, with or without a palpable mass or signs of ascites, may be present. Pelvic examination will often reveal an ovarian mass. The chest should be assessed for pleural effusion and the lymph nodes in the neck palpated for distant nodal spread.

Investigations

Routine haematological and biochemical tests are usually normal. A chest radiograph may demonstrate metastases or pleural effusion. Imaging of the abdomen and pelvis is essential; ultrasound is particularly good at imaging the ovaries and identifying ovarian cysts and the presence of ascites. CT scan of the abdomen and pelvis will also demonstrate the primary tumour and the presence of any pelvic or paraortic enlargement. However CT scanning often underestimates the amount of disease in the omentum and around the bowel. Serum CA 125 is a useful blood marker for ovarian cancer which is elevated in 80% of cases, particularly in those with serous histology, and is a useful monitor of response to treatment.

Staging

Ovarian cancer is staged using the FIGO system as shown in Table 11.3.

Treatment

A tissue diagnosis is essential and a laparotomy should be performed. The abdomen should be opened with a vertical incision to allow adequate inspection of all peritoneal surfaces and intra-abdominal organs. A total abdominal hysterectomy, bilateral salpingo-oophorectomy and removal of the omentum should be performed

---

Stage I
Confined to the ovary
a One ovary involved
b Both ovaries involved
c Associated malignant ascites

Stage II
Spread within the pelvis

Stage III
Spread to the abdominal cavity

Stage IV
Distant metastases

Table 11.3   FIGO staging for cancer of the ovary

and any metastases identified debulked if possible. The smaller the amount of residual disease remaining at the end of surgery the better the prognosis. The amount of debulking achieved depends on the biology of the tumour as well as the skill of the surgeon. However, increasingly, specialist gynaecological surgeons are undertaking these operations to increase the possibility of maximal debulking.

Post-operative treatment

The optimum post-operative treatment for patients with stage I disease is unknown. Those with well-differentiated stage I disease without ascites or adhesion to neighbouring organs have an excellent prognosis, probably requiring no further treatment. However, those with poorly differentiated disease, particularly in the presence of ascites, cyst rupture or adherence to neighbouring structures have a relapse rate up to 30% and may benefit from adjuvant chemotherapy. The role of adjuvant chemotherapy is currently being tested in an international clinical trial.

For more advanced disease, chemotherapy is routine. Cisplatin or carboplatin are the usual drugs, used typically as single agents in the UK, but as part of combination chemotherapy in other parts of Europe and the USA. The response rate to platinum agents is 60–70%. Carboplatin is generally preferred as it is considerably less toxic, causing less nausea and vomiting, neurotoxicity, nephrotoxicity and ototoxicity although bone marrow suppression is more pronounced. The drug does not require intensive hydration and can be given on an out-patient basis. The results have been identical to those achieved with the older analogue cisplatin.

Alternatively, single alkylating agent therapy can be used and is often preferred for elderly or frail patients. It has little toxicity and although the response rate is only about 30%, patients who fail to respond to alkylating agent therapy or who relapse afterwards may be salvaged by platinum-containing regimens.

Recently, a new highly active drug, paclitaxel (Taxol), has been introduced for the management of ovarian cancer. For the first time a significant number of patients with platinum resistance have shown responses to treatment and preliminary studies suggest a combination of Taxol and platinum is better than previous combination chemotherapy regimens.

For patients in whom surgical debulking is not possible, a second operation in those patients showing response to chemotherapy appears to improve the prognosis compared with giving chemotherapy alone.

Radiotherapy is rarely indicated in the management of ovarian cancer. The previous enthusiasm for wide field irradiation of the pelvis and abdomen has largely disappeared in most centres. Radiotherapy may be of value for palliation of symptomatic recurrent pelvic masses, vaginal bleeding or painful bone disease.

Prognosis

Patients with stage I ovarian cancer have a good prognosis with 80% 5-year survival. For more advanced disease, the results are considerably worse. Patients with stage III disease have a 30% 5-year survival and fewer than 5% of patients with stage IV disease will survive 5 years.

Patients who relapse after primary chemotherapy may be re-treated with the same drugs if they have shown response for at least a year. For those showing resistance to platinum or relapsing within 12 months, chemotherapy, other than perhaps pacli-taxel, is unhelpful.

Other tumours of the ovary

Clear cell carcinoma of the ovary is generally managed in the same way as other epithelial tumours but has a more variable pattern of metastases and responds less predictably to chemotherapy. Brenner tumours (fibromas) are almost always benign and typically slow growing. Surgical removal is indicated. Germ cell tumours should be removed surgically and chemotherapy based on the extent of disease and pres-ence of elevated tumour markers (AFP and β-HCG). Patients with evidence of active disease should receive combination chemotherapy as used for testicular tumours. The prognosis is generally excellent.

Granulosa cell tumours are of low grade and usually cured surgically. However metastases do occur, often years later. The tumour may secrete oestrogens. Palliation of advanced disease with chemotherapy is possible.

Rarely, sarcomas and mixed mesodermal tumours showing both sarcomatous and epithelial elements arise in the ovary. The prognosis is usually poor even though responses to chemotherapy are quite commonly seen.

Metastases in the ovary are quite common, particularly from tumours arising in the stomach or breast cancer. Historically, ovarian metastases from carcinoma of the stomach have been referred to as Krukenberg tumours.

Vagina

Carcinoma of the vagina is very uncommon, causing fewer than 150 deaths a year in the UK. It is usually a disease of elderly women although cases in young women or children have been reported, related to oestrogen therapy in the mother during pregnancy and lactation. Most primary carcinomas of the vagina are of a squamous cell type, sometimes associated with the long-term use of ring pessaries.

The tumour spreads locally and also via the lymphatics. This is to pelvic and para-aortic lymph nodes from upper vaginal lesions and to the groin nodes from those arising lower in the vagina.

Typically the disease presents with bleeding and the lesion can usually be clearly seen on inspection.

In young women, the disease is best treated by radical surgery while for those who are older or less fit, radical radiotherapy with external beam radiation and intracavitary treatment are recommended.

Vulva

Cancer of the vulva is also uncommon. Again, most carcinomas are of squamous type, usually occurring in old age. They may be associated with chronic irritative conditions of the vulval skin. Leucoplakia, lichen sclerosis, Paget's disease of the vulva and carcinoma *in situ* are all pre-malignant conditions. Typically the lesion presents with pruritus followed by thickening of the vulval skin, which may then ulcerate and bleed. Bilateral tumours may occur. As with vaginal carcinoma, local invasion is the principal problem, plus lymphatic spread to the inguinal and iliac lymph nodes. Blood-borne spread is a late event.

Treatment is generally surgical with radical vulvectomy plus bilateral block dissection of the lymph nodes. Radiotherapy may be used as an alternative in patients who are unfit for surgery, but the vulval skin is relatively intolerant to radiation. Small lesions may be treated with radioactive needle implants. Sometimes chemotherapy with mitomycin C and fluorouracil is recommended for palliation of recurrent or extensive disease with occasional benefit.

In general, the prognosis is quite good for those who are able to withstand radical surgery with 80% of patients alive at 5 years.

Gestational trophoblastic disease

Trophoblastic tissue can undergo progressive cellular changes from simple hydropic degeneration, through hydatidiform mole and invasive mole to choriocarcinoma. In the UK, hydatidiform moles occur in about 1 in 700 pregnancies and choriocarcinoma in 1 in 30 000. However, the incidence of the latter is much higher in Asia. Choriocarcinoma usually arises as a complication of hydatidiform mole, but in about 25% of cases occurs after a normal or ectopic pregnancy.

Local growth is rapid and metastases arise early, usually in the lungs but also sometimes in the brain. The tumour tissue invariably produces HCG and estimation of the β subunit in the urine or serum is of diagnostic and prognostic value.

The disease generally presents as abnormal vaginal bleeding within 1 year of pregnancy. Abdominal or pelvic discomfort may be present, and occasionally patients will have symptoms of metastatic disease. Pelvic examination may reveal an enlarged and tender uterus; chest signs secondary to pulmonary metastases occur late.

Management

Gestational trophoblastic disease is managed in the UK by three supra-regional units in London, Sheffield and Dundee. Any patient developing a hydatidiform mole should be registered with one of these centres, which will organize screening of urine samples for production of HCG. In most women, gestational trophoblastic disease will resolve spontaneously following curettage of the uterus. However in about 5–6% of patients the disease persists, despite a second or third uterine curettage, and chemotherapy becomes necessary. The indications for chemotherapy include: a histological diagnosis of choriocarcinoma; very high (>20 000 i.u./l) or rising HCG levels after curettage; persistently elevated levels more than 6 months after curettage; troublesome vaginal bleeding; and evidence of widespread or very bulky metastatic disease.

Investigations

All patients requiring chemotherapy are staged with serum levels of β-HCG, examination of the pelvis and radiological assessment of the chest. From this information a prognostic score can be calculated and chemotherapy will be based on this.

For patients with a good prognosis, single agent, intramuscular methotrexate is a highly effective agent and will cure 85% of such patients. For the 15% of patients with good prognosis who fail to respond to methotrexate, salvage is invariably possible with a combination of etoposide and actinomycin D. Patients who fall into the poor prognostic category can usually be cured with a combination of high-dose methotrexate, etoposide and actinomycin D. Despite the label of poor prognosis the end results are generally excellent with a cure rate in excess of 98%.

After successful treatment many women go on to have further pregnancies without complications. There is, however, an increased risk of a subsequent molar pregnancy in those with a previous history of trophoblastic disease.

12

Cancer of the male genital tract

R E COLEMAN

Testis

Testicular tumours account for only 1% of all cancers but are the most common malignancy in young men aged 18–35 years. In the UK, there are just over 1000 cases per year and the incidence is rising quite steeply. There are two main types of testicular tumour. Seminoma is the most common type occurring in 50% of patients with a peak incidence in the fourth decade of life, while teratomas occur in a third of patients with peak incidence in the third decade of life. Most of the remaining tumours are a mixture of both seminoma and teratoma. There are a number of other very rare tumours of the testis including Leydig cell tumours, lymphomas and sarcomas.

Testicular tumours are thought to arise as a developmental abnormality and are much more common in men with a history of testicular maldescent. Bilateral tumours develop in around 3%.

Pathology

Seminomas are solid tumours which are generally well circumscribed with a pale lobulated appearance, whereas teratomas are usually haemorrhagic and contain cysts. Microscopically, seminomas are fairly uniform tumours. Particularly well-differentiated varieties are recognized (spermatocytic seminomas). Teratomas may contain a range of cell types with varying differentiation. They may be completely undifferentiated or show elements of either trophoblastic differentiation or yolk sac tissue.

Testicular tumours invade locally into the tunica vaginalis and along the spermatic cord. Seminomas spread predominantly via the lymphatic system to para-aortic and mediastinal lymph nodes while teratomas metastasize both to lymph nodes and via the blood mainly to the lungs but also the liver and brain.

Symptoms and signs

Testicular swelling or discomfort is the most common presenting sign but backache from enlarged para-aortic lymph nodes and cough, haemoptysis or dyspnoea from

1 Limited to the testis
2 Involving lymph nodes below the diaphragm
3 Involving lymph nodes both sides of the diaphragm
4 Distant metastases (L) lungs, (H) liver

Further sub-division of stages is made on the basis of tumour bulk and number of lung metastases

Table 12.1   Royal Marsden staging of testicular cancer

lung metastases may be reported. Occasionally the testicular swelling may regress spontaneously, leaving a small scar which may only be identifiabie on ultrasound examination. Clinically a testicular swelling may have an associated hydrocele and patients with extensive lymph node disease may have a palpable central abdominal mass.

Investigations

In all patients with a testicular tumour, measurement of specific serum markers for germ cell tumours should be performed before surgery and regularly thereafter during follow-up. The two important serum markers are AFP and β-HCG. Placental alkaline phosphatase (PLAP) is of some value for monitoring patients with seminoma, but is also affected by cigarette smoking. About 90% of patients with a teratoma will have either AFP or β-HCG elevated and 40–50% will have both markers raised. β-HCG may be elevated in patients with seminoma while AFP elevation always indicates teratomatous elements.

All patients should be staged with a CT scan of the pelvis, abdomen and chest to evaluate pelvic lymph nodes and identify lung metastases. A CT scan of the brain should be performed in patients with very extensive disease particularly if they have a trophoblastic tumour with very high levels of β-HCG. Testicular tumours are most commonly staged in the UK using the Royal Marsden Hospital staging system (Table 12.1).

Treatment

The initial treatment of all testicular tumours is orchidectomy. This removes the primary tumour and provides the pathologist with the best possible material for an accurate histological diagnosis. This should be performed through an inguinal incision. An orchidectomy performed through the scrotum runs a risk of tumour implantation in the wound and subsequent local relapse.

Treatment after orchidectomy depends on the result of staging tests. In those patients with a normal staging CT scan and return of tumour markers to normal (stage I disease) the prognosis is extremely good with about 75% of teratomas and 85% of seminomas cured without further treatment.

Because seminomas are exquisitely radiosensitive, many centres recommend adjuvant radiotherapy to the para-aortic lymph nodes and ipsilateral pelvic nodes. A relatively low dose is usually sufficient. Alternatively, patients with seminoma can be watched carefully with regular follow-up CT scans and tumour marker estimations to detect recurrence which can almost always be salvaged by further treatment at that time. This approach avoids irradiation for the majority of patients who do not need it and, because a large area of bone marrow has not been irradiated, the administration of chemotherapy to those patients who do subsequently relapse is less hazardous.

For patients with stage I teratoma, intensive surveillance is the usually recommended management in Europe. Tumour markers are assessed monthly and abdominal and chest CT scans performed every 3–4 months during the first 2 years of follow-up. Alternatively, those with poor prognosis stage I disease with certain histological features, particularly vascular invasion, may be offered a short course of adjuvant chemotherapy.

Patients with more extensive disease usually require chemotherapy. For those with teratoma the choice of chemotherapy depends on various prognostic factors. For the majority of patients with good prognosis, standard chemotherapy with four 3-weekly cycles of BEP (bleomycin, etoposide and cisplatin) will cure 85–90% of patients. High-risk patients with very extensive disease, liver or brain involvement and grossly elevated markers (AFP >1000 or β-HCG >10 000) should probably receive more intensive regimens using alternating drug schedules administered every 7–10 days.

Patients with advanced seminoma are usually also treated with chemotherapy except in those with very small para-aortic lymph nodes (stage IIa). These patients can be treated effectively by radiotherapy alone to the para-aortic and pelvic lymph nodes. All other patients receive four courses of cisplatin and etoposide with most showing an excellent long-term response to this treatment.

After chemotherapy, all patients should be reassessed for evidence of residual disease. In some cases a residual mass will be seen, despite normalization of tumour markers. If these masses persist for more than a few months they should be removed surgically. Although many will show only necrosis and cystic degeneration, others will show differentiated teratoma which with time can de-differentiate to a malignant phenotype and subsequent relapse. In addition, a small focus of malignant cells may be found in the resected specimen despite normal tumour markers. This surgery is often difficult and requires specialized surgical expertise.

Overall, the prognosis of testicular tumours is excellent, even patients with very extensive lung involvement or liver or brain metastases can be cured. For patients relapsing on surveillance, cure is expected in more than 95% of patients while about 85% of those with more advanced stages are cured. Relapse is most common in the first 12–18 months after diagnosis or chemotherapy but occasional late relapses are seen and the risk of second tumours should not be overlooked.

Prostate

Carcinoma of the prostate is a disease primarily of elderly men. The incidence is increasing with about 12 000 cases a year in the UK and 10% of cancer deaths. The disease is rare under the age of 45 years and increases in incidence to become almost a universal post-mortem finding in men dying over the age of 85. In young men with the disease there may also be a positive family history. Benign prostatic hypertrophy is often also present but there is no definite relationship between the development of benign hypertrophy and malignant change.

Pathology

Prostate tumours are typically adenocarcinomas developing most frequently in the outer part of the gland, often with a multifocal origin. Histological grading of the tumour is usually performed as this gives prognostic information. Positive staining of the tumour is usually seen for acid phosphatase and prostate specific antigen (PSA).

Screening

Screening for prostate cancer is being extensively evaluated using one or more of a combination of digital rectal examination, trans-rectal ultrasound and serum measurement of PSA. Screening undoubtedly leads to earlier detection of the cancer but whether this affects the quality and quantity of survival in these generally elderly men is at present unknown.

Symptoms and signs

Prostate cancer may present in various ways. Symptoms of urinary outflow obstruction are most common with frequency, poor stream, nocturia and dribbling of urine. In some cases, the disease presents with symptoms of bone metastases with bone pain or cord compression while in others the disease may be asymptomatic and found incidentally during investigation of another condition or at post mortem.

The disease spreads by both local infiltration into surrounding tissues and via the bloodstream, particularly through the vertebral plexus of veins to the skeleton. Bone is by far the most common metastatic site affected. Occasionally lymph node metastases and soft tissue metastases in the lung or liver may occur but these are rarely a clinical problem.

Rectal examination may reveal the tumour as a hard nodule or a diffusely infiltrated enlarged prostate. Usually the mid-line sulcus is lost while in the normal or hypertrophied prostate this is preserved.

Investigations

Patients with prostate cancer should be investigated with routine blood tests to check for anaemia and bone marrow infiltration and renal function which may be affected by ureteric obstruction. Serum should be sent for measurement of PSA and in addition serum acid phosphatase can be helpful.

An isotope bone scan is the investigation of choice to identify bone metastases. Imaging of the pelvis by ultrasound or CT will give additional information on the local extent of disease. Diagnosis is made by histology obtained either via trans-urethral resection of the prostate (TURP) or by a needle biopsy performed through the rectal mucosa. The latter is preferred unless there are urinary symptoms that require surgical intervention.

Staging investigations are important to identify whether the disease is a co-incidental finding (stage A), confined within the capsule of the gland (stage B), locally advanced (stage C) or associated with metastases (stage D).

Treatment

For patients with localized disease, the choice of treatment is between radical prostatectomy and radical radiotherapy. The surgery is technically difficult and many patients subsequently experience impotence. Potency is not usually affected by radical radiotherapy but bladder and bowel toxicity may occur.

Most patients with recurrent or metastatic disease achieve a temporary response with hormone therapy. A number of endocrine treatments are possible including surgical orchidectomy, low-dose oestrogens, androgens and, more recently, the gonadotrophin-releasing hormone (GnRH) agonists. GnRH treatment prevents the release of gonadotrophins from the pituitary and results in low levels of testosterone similar to those achieved after surgical castration. However, in the first week or two of treatment a temporary flare in testosterone levels and worsening of symptoms may occur. Many specialists recommend the use of additional anti-androgen drugs during this period.

After an initial response to endocrine therapy, relapse is inevitable with the average duration of response being around 18 months. Second responses to hormones occasionally occur but eventually the disease becomes hormone resistant. Chemotherapy is rarely effective and generally too toxic for this elderly population. For patients with bone metastases, sensible prescription of analgesics, local or wide-field radiotherapy, bone-seeking radioisotopes and bisphosphonates may all help in palliation.

Penis

Malignant disease of the penis is rare and is almost always a squamous cell carcinoma. Incidence is high in certain parts of Asia and rarely recorded in males circumcised as infants. There may be a viral aetiology. The disease usually affects the elderly. Most tumours arise in the glans but occasionally develop on the shaft. Surgical management is usually recommended except for local lesions and in patients wishing to continue sexual activity. As an alternative, radical radiotherapy can provide an effective treatment modality. Because lymphatic spread is to the inguinal lymph nodes, radical block dissection or local radiotherapy to the inguinal regions may be needed. In the absence of lymph node metastases the prognosis is good.

13

Cancer of the urinary tract

R E COLEMAN

Kidney

Renal cell carcinoma (hypernephroma) is the usual malignant tumour of the kidney in adults. There are nearly 4000 cases each year in the UK with men affected slightly more frequently than women. The disease is most common in the sixth and seventh decades of life. Renal cell carcinomas arise from the epithelium of the renal tubules, but apart from a relationship with smoking, little is known about aetiological factors.

Pathology

Histologically these tumours are adenocarcinomas composed of cells with characteristically clear cytoplasm showing variable differentiation.

Local extension of the tumour into the renal vein and then on into the inferior vena cava is common. Usually the tumour is solid, expanding the renal tissue with central necrosis or cystic degeneration and haemorrhage. The tumour invades the surrounding kidney and may spread via the lymph nodes to the renal hilar lymph nodes and para-aortic lymph node chain or via the bloodstream to the lung and bone particularly, but also on occasions the skin and CNS.

Symptoms and signs

Typically the tumour grows without symptoms until locally advanced or until distant metastases are present, for example a pathological fracture through a bone deposit. However, some present early, usually with haematuria, loin pain or episodes of pyrexia. Rarely, the tumour is associated with polycythaemia due to erythropoietin production.

Examination of the patient may reveal a palpable mass in the loin and about 15% of patients have associated fever.

Investigations

Investigations should include a full blood count which may show polycythaemia. Urea, electrolyte and creatinine measurements are essential. Microscopy of urine for red blood cells and a chest X-ray for lung metastases may be helpful. The tumour is usually well visualized by ultrasound which will also facilitate a tissue diagnosis by fine needle aspiration cytology or biopsy. CT scanning will give additional information on involvement of the renal bed or extension into the renal vein. A bone scan may reveal metastases but as these are typically lytic they may be missed by radionuclide bone scanning. Plain radiographs should therefore be performed if there is clinical suspicion of bone involvement.

Treatment

Surgery is the only curative treatment and where possible radical nephrectomy should be performed, with care taken to remove any tumour invading the renal vein. Some centres recommend pre-operative arterial embolization of large tumours. This may facilitate subsequent surgery but probably has no effect on eventual outcome. Post-operative radiotherapy to the renal bed may improve the local control of locally advanced tumours but is inadequate treatment on its own.

The systemic management of renal cell carcinoma is difficult. Very occasionally, spontaneous regression of metastases has been recorded after removal of the primary tumour while a few patients (10%) may show response to hormone therapy with progestogens. Chemotherapy is ineffective but in recent years biological agents, such as IFN and IL-2, have been shown to induce remissions, particularly in lung and lymph node metastases, in about 15–20% of patients. Current research is likely to define the true place of these expensive and sometimes toxic agents.

Finally, renal cell cancer is sometimes associated with solitary metastases either in lung, brain or bone. It is one of the few epithelial tumours in which surgical excision of a metastatic lesion can be recommended.

The prognosis of renal cell carcinoma is relatively good with 50% of patients surviving 5 years. Even patients with metastases may have a long and indolent natural history with a few surviving more than 5 years.

Other tumours of the kidney and urinary collecting system

These are rare tumours usually of transitional cell type occurring most commonly in men. They may be multifocal and, when operable, surgical excision is the treatment of choice.

In children, nephroblastoma (Wilms' tumour) is an important malignancy which is discussed in Chapter 15.

Bladder

Malignant tumours of the bladder generally affect elderly men in their seventies and eighties. About 10 000 cases are seen in the UK each year. They rarely present before the age of 50 and affect twice as many men as women.

TIS		*In situ* carcinoma
T1		Superficial carcinoma without muscle involvement
T2		Invasion of superficial muscle
T3		Invasion of deep muscle
	a	Within the bladder wall
	b	Into perivesical fat
T4		Extravesical spread
	a	Invasion of neighbouring pelvic structures
	b	Distant metastases

Table 13.1   TNM staging of bladder cancer

A variety of aetiological factors have been identified. These include chemical carcinogens including aniline dyes and byproducts from the rubber industry such as β-naphthylamine and exposure to drugs like phenacetin or cyclophosphamide. Smoking is also an important aetiological factor due to excretion of carcinogenic tar products from absorbed tobacco smoke. Bladder cancer may be precipitated by chronic irritation of the mucosa within diverticula or from calculi or in some parts of the world, particularly Egypt, by schistosomiasis.

Pathology

Bladder cancers usually develop as papillomas which if untreated will progress to invasive carcinoma. They are often multiple and may vary histologically through all grades from well-differentiated (G1) to poorly differentiated anaplastic (G3) tumours. More than 90% of bladder cancers are transitional cell carcinomas, except in Egypt where the schistosomiasis-related tumour is typically squamous cell in type.

Bladder cancers most frequently affect the base and lateral walls of the bladder invading locally into the muscle and then into perivesical fat. Spread is both via the lymph nodes in the pelvis and para-aortic region and the bloodstream particularly to the lungs and bone.

Bladder cancer is usually staged using TNM staging system as shown in Table 13.1.

Symptoms and signs

The most important presenting symptom of bladder cancer is painless haematuria which always merits serious investigation. Frequency, urgency and dysuria may also be present. Other symptoms and physical signs are unusual unless the disease is widespread.

Investigations

These should include cytological examination of the urine which may reveal malignant cells and cystoscopy. During cystoscopy, the entire mucosal surface can be assessed and biopsies taken of abnormal areas. In addition, transurethral resection of bladder tumours may be performed at the same time.

In patients with invasive disease, when cystectomy is under consideration, a CT scan should be performed to assess extravesical extension of tumour and lymph node enlargement. An intravenous urogram may demonstrate a filling defect in the bladder but is more useful in that it helps to exclude tumours in other parts of the urinary tract.

Treatment

Small superficial well-differentiated tumours, whether single or multiple, are best treated by transurethral resection. This should be followed by careful and frequent cystoscopic examination so that any recurrence or new tumours can be detected early and treated. Multiple tumours may require several sessions of treatment. Recurrence will occur in about one-half of patients and progression of disease with more invasion and worsening histological features is also seen in 15–20% of patients.

Intravesical chemotherapy is useful for controlling superficial bladder cancer. A variety of agents including mitomycin C, doxorubicin, thiotepa and BCG have all been used to good effect.

For progressive, invasive disease the choice is between radiotherapy and cystectomy. Radical radiotherapy allows the patient to retain the bladder but many patients will either not respond adequately to radiotherapy or subsequently progress. Radiotherapy to the bladder also causes unpleasant acute symptoms with urinary frequency, dysuria, diarrhoea and tenesmus and often results in a shrunken, fibrosed bladder. Cystectomy is a major operation which many of these elderly patients will be unable to withstand. However, for those who are fit, elective cystectomy with or without additional radiotherapy is preferred by many centres.

For those with locally advanced tumours or who are too frail to tolerate radical treatment, palliative radiotherapy will help relieve bladder symptoms, particularly haematuria and pain. Although transitional cell carcinoma is a relatively chemosensitive tumour the role of chemotherapy in routine management has yet to be defined. The most widely used drug combination is cisplatin, methotrexate and vinblastine with responses in about one-half of patients treated.

The prognosis of bladder cancer is very stage dependent, ranging from 70% for T1 tumours, 50% for T2, 20% for T3 and less than 10% for T4 tumours. Because of the instability of the transitional epithelium in some patients the possibility of a new primary developing elsewhere in the urothelial system should always be kept in mind.

Urethra

Malignant tumours of the urethra are rare. They may be either transitional cell or squamous in type. They are managed in much the same way as bladder tumours. However, in women, a urostomy will usually be required and therefore a radioactive needle implant may provide a more acceptable effective alternative.

14

Myeloproliferative and lymphoproliferative disorders

P C LORIGAN and B W HANCOCK

The malignancies derived from cells of the bone marrow and lymphoreticular system comprise mainly the leukaemias, the lymphomas and myeloma (Table 14.1). These neoplasms account for less than 10% of all malignant disease, but are important, because many are now known to be curable by the newer techniques of radiotherapy and cytotoxic chemotherapy. Modern treatment has greatly improved the prognosis in this group of tumours. Some are now potentially curable, whereas 30 years ago they would have been fatal.

Leukaemias
Acute
   Acute lymphoblastic leukaemia (ALL)
   Acute myeloid leukaemia (AML)
Chronic
   Chronic lymphocytic leukaemia (CLL)
   Chronic myeloid leukaemia (CML)

Lymphomas
   Hodgkin's disease
   Non-Hodgkin's lymphoma
     Low grade
     Intermediate/high grade

Multiple myeloma

Other disorders
Myeloproliferative
   Myelofibrosis
   Polycythaemia rubra vera
Lymphoproliferative
   Waldenstrom's macroglobulinaemia
   Heavy chain disease
   Hairy cell leukaemia

Table 14.1 Malignancies derived from cells of the bone marrow and lymphoreticular system

Acute leukaemia

Acute lymphoblastic leukaemia (ALL) is the most common leukaemia in childhood, and acute myeloid leukaemia (AML) is the most common leukaemia in adults.

Genetic factors are important in aetiology. There is a lower incidence of ALL in black children, a higher incidence in identical twins with an affected sibling and an increased incidence with certain inherited conditions, such as Down's syndrome and Fanconi's anaemia. Exposure to radiation and certain chemicals (e.g. benzene) increases the risk. Previous treatment with chemotherapy greatly increases the risk. Certain viruses have also been implicated, for example human T lymphotrophic virus type 1 (HTLV-1), causes a rare but very aggressive form of leukaemia. Paternal exposure to radiation and exposure to electromagnetic fields have not yet been proved to be aetiological factors.

The history is usually short and may be non-specific with general malaise. Other symptoms include anaemia, bruising and bleeding due to thrombocytopenia or disseminated intravascular coagulation (DIC), bone pain, enlarging lymphadenopathy, infection and symptoms of hyperviscosity. Lymphadenopathy and splenomegaly are more common in ALL, hyperviscosity is usually confined to AML.

The diagnosis is usually made by examination of the bone marrow and studying the peripheral blood film. Samples should be taken for cytogenetic and immunocytochemistry analysis.

Acute lymphoblastic leukaemia

Several classification systems exist and a combination of methods is often used. The lymphoblasts may be classified by morphology using the FAB classification system (French, American, British), into three subgroups L1–L3, with ALL L3 having the worst prognosis. However, distinguishing lymphoblasts morphologically can be difficult. Alternatively, immunocytochemistry can be used to define cell-surface markers. Phenotype correlates with prognosis. Using this classification, lymphoblasts are classified as being common ALL, B cell ALL, T cell ALL or null ALL.

The following pre-treatment factors are associated with a poor prognosis: high white cell count; male sex (the testis is a sanctuary site for leukaemia); CNS involvement; age less than 2 years or greater than 20 years; and black race. Morphological, immunocytochemical and cytogenetic factors give added prognostic information.

Acute myeloid leukaemia

There are seven subgroups (M1–M7) of AML. Of particular importance is acute promyelocytic leukaemia (M3), which may present with DIC. It has a high initial mortality but a better long-term survival after successful remission than other types. Acute monocytic leukaemia (M5) is associated with gum hypertrophy and renal tubular loss of potassium.

Treatment of acute leukaemia

Treatment of ALL consists of a number of phases: inducing remission; CNS prophylaxis; maintenance therapy or ablative therapy and haematological rescue.

Remission is achieved in over 80% of patients with a combination of drugs, including prednisolone, daunorubicin and vincristine. These drugs will cause a period of bone marrow suppression during which time patients will require intensive medical supervision, blood and platelet support and antibiotics. The cerebrospinal fluid (CSF), a sanctuary site, should be examined for leukaemic infiltration once the blood is clear of blasts. Following successful remission, CNS prophylaxis with either high-dose methotrexate and/or craniospinal irradiation should be carried out. This may then be followed by a period of intensification using combination chemotherapy. Following this, maintenance treatment for up to 2 years with oral cytotoxics is usually advised. For patients with poor prognostic factors who are at high risk of relapse, further high-dose chemotherapy with haematological rescue may be considered (see below).

Treatment of AML consists of: inducing remission; consolidation of remission; ablative therapy for younger patients or high-dose oral chemotherapy for older patients.

Remission is achieved by using a combination of drugs, including daunorubicin, cytosine and thioguanine, in about 75% of cases. This is followed by two further courses of this treatment to consolidate this remission. Consideration is then given to high-dose chemotherapy.

High-dose chemotherapy

Although most patients with acute leukaemia achieve remission, many relapse due to the presence of occult disease that has not been eradicated. High-dose chemotherapy can eradicate this occult disease, but at the expense of irreversible damage to the bone marrow stem cells. To circumvent this problem, bone marrow can be removed either from the patient or from a human leucocyte antigen (HLA) compatible donor, stored and then re-infused after high-dose chemotherapy to replace the damaged bone marrow.

In autologous bone marrow transplantation (ABMT), there is a very real risk that the re-infused bone marrow will itself contain malignant cells. There are a number of ways to minimize this risk (see below).

In an allogenic bone marrow transplant, the bone marrow is harvested from an HLA compatible donor, usually a sibling, but occasionally a matched but completely unrelated donor. There is no risk of malignant contamination of the donor bone marrow. The donor bone marrow will recognize any residual leukaemia as foreign and destroy it (graft *versus* leukaemia). Unfortunately, the donor bone marrow may also see the recipient as foreign and attack this (i.e. graft *versus* host disease; GVHD). This may be acute and is characterized by skin changes, multisystem failure and possibly death. Chronic GVHD is characterized by chronic inflammatory changes which may affect many organs. GVHD is minimized by the use of immunosuppressants, namely cyclosporin A, methotrexate and steroids. These drugs have their own side-effects and prolonged immunosuppression can result in opportunistic, often lethal, infections and secondary malignancies.

There have been some new developments in treatment. Bone marrow purging is one example. It can be effected by a number of methods. The bone marrow can be grown *in vitro* for about 10 days, during which time the fastidious leukaemic cells die off. Alternatively the pluripotent stem cells can be selectively harvested from the bone marrow and this sample then treated with complement and antibodies to kill malignant cells.

In another development, patients are treated with chemotherapy and/or growth factors which causes the release of progenitor cells into the peripheral blood. These peripheral blood stem cells (PBSC) can be easily harvested and used for haemopoietic rescue. They engraft in about half the time of bone marrow and reduce the risk of malignant contamination. High-dose chemotherapy and PBSC rescue will probably soon replace high-dose chemotherapy and ABMT.

Differentiation therapy is another new development. Acute promyelocytic leukaemia (M3) is characterized by the t(15;17) translocation, with the break point on chromosome 17 being at the retinoic acid receptor gene. Treatment of M3 AML with retinoic acid results in differentiation of the malignant promyelocytes into mature myeloid cells. Chemotherapy is eventually required owing to the development of drug resistance, but this is an elective setting, without the 20% risk of death due to haemorrhagic complications.

Chronic leukaemia

Chronic myeloid leukaemia

Chronic myeloid leukaemia (CML) is a relatively uncommon form of leukaemia which occurs most commonly in people aged 30–60 years.

The clinical presentation is classically that of splenomegaly with its associated symptoms, or chronic ill health with anaemia and bleeding problems. It may be a chance finding.

The diagnosis is established by finding a raised peripheral white cell count, often greater than $50 \times 10^9/l$, consisting mainly of myelocytes, neutrophils and blasts. Cytogenetics show the classical Philadelphia chromosome t(9;22) translocation (i.e. reciprocal translocation of the long arm of chromosome 22 to chromosome 9). This results in the transposition of the *BCR* gene to a site beside the *ABL* gene. The leucocyte alkaline phosphatase is greatly reduced.

Treatment is usually with busulfan or hydroxyurea, the latter may be given in high-dose pulses to get the malignant cells into the cell cycle and destroy them while minimizing toxicity to stem cells. Irradiation of the spleen can be considered, to reduce pain and alleviate anaemia and thrombocytopenia.

After 3–4 years, a blast cell crisis occurs and the condition transforms into acute leukaemia (usually AML, but very occasionally ALL). Survival after blast transformation is poor, but trials of high-dose chemotherapy and PBSC/ABMT are underway.

Chronic lymphocytic leukaemia

Chronic lymphocytic leukaemia (CLL) is a disease of the late middle aged and elderly. The onset is usually insidious with lethargy, fever and weight loss. It may be a coincidental finding. Physical signs are of generalized lymphadenopathy with or without hepatosplenomegaly. The peripheral white cell count may be very high ($>100 \times 10^9$/l). Most of these are clonal B lymphocytes. There may be haemolytic anaemia and there is a reduction in humoral immunity.

Staging is with the Rai and Binet staging system (Table 14.2). Higher stages have a poorer prognosis.

Treatment is palliative with alkylating agents, such as chlorambucil or cyclophosphamide. Newer purine analogues (e.g. fludarabine) may become the treatment of choice. Experimental treatments include the use of other purine analogues, such as 2-chlorodeoxyadenosine, or humanized monoclonal antibodies. Prognosis is good, with median survival over 10 years. Patients are often elderly and die of other causes.

Malignant lymphoma

Malignant lymphoma is divided into two groups of disease: Hodgkin's disease and non-Hodgkin's lymphoma. The former has a fairly well standardized histology typing, staging criteria and treatment protocols; the latter is a much more heterogeneous group of conditions with a wide variety of histological types, staging classifications and treatment protocols. Some contrasting features can be identified (Table 14.3).

Hodgkin's disease

Hodgkin's disease is the most common lymphoma in the Western world. Its incidence is 3.4 per 100 000 per year and is falling. There is a bimodal peak age incidence, one peak occurring at 15–34 years and the other after 50 years. There is a slight male preponderance. The aetiology is unknown but there is mounting evidence to implicate EBV in at least one of the subtypes.

Two-thirds of cases present with cervical lymphadenopathy, although any lymph node group or extranodal site may be involved. Patients may also complain of high swinging temperatures, drenching sweats and weight loss of more than 10% of their body weight. Other symptoms may include pruritus, alcohol-induced pain and a variety of other constitutional symptoms.

A number of non-specific findings are commonly found, including anaemia or raised ESR. Diagnosis is established by demonstrating histological evidence of Hodgkin's disease in a biopsy, usually of a lymph node. The malignant cell is felt to be the characteristic bi-nucleate Reed–Sternberg cell.

There are four main histological subtypes of Hodgkin's disease in the Rai classification: lymphocyte predominant; nodular sclerosing; mixed cellularity; and lymphocyte depleted.

Stage	Lymphocytosis	Lymphadenopathy	Splenomegaly or hepatomegaly	Haemoglobin (g/dl)	Platelets ($\times 10^9/1$)
0	+	–	–	>11	>100
1	+	+	–	>11	>100
2	+	±	+	>11	>100
3	+	±	±	<11	>100
4	+	±	±	<11	<100
Binet system					
A	+	± (<3 lymphatic groups positive)	±	≥10	≥100
B	+	± (<3 lymphatic groups positive)	±	≥10	≥100
C	+	±	±	>10	>100

Table 14.2 Rai staging classification

Feature	Hodgkin's disease	Non-Hodgkin's lymphoma
Age	Younger	Older
Male:female ratio	3:2	6:5
Presentation	Neck nodes most common	Unusual nodes or extranodal sites; often generalized
Histology	Rai classification	High *versus* low grade
Spread	Contiguous (unifocal origin)	Generalized (multifocal origin)
Treatment	Localized: radiotherapy	Usually 'symptomatic' for low grade and intensive chemotherapy for high grade
	Others: cyclical chemotherapy with or without radiotherapy	
Prognosis	Over two-thirds of patients are cured	Low grade: median survival 7–8 years (rarely cured)
		High grade: over one-third of patients are cured

Table 14.3 Contrasting features of Hodgkin's disease and non-Hodgkin's lymphoma

Stage 1	Single lymph node region involved
Stage 2	Two or more lymph node regions involved but on the same side of the diaphragm
Stage 3	Involvement of lymph node regions on both sides of the diaphragm
Stage 4	Generalized involvement of one or more extralymphatic organs with or without lymph node disease

Localized extralymphatic lesions with or without associated lymph node involvement are termed E (extranodal) lesions

Category A	Asymptomatic
Category B	Symptomatic (night sweats and/or weight loss and/or fever)

Table 14.4   Ann Arbor staging criteria

Staging

Staging is by the Ann Arbor (Table 14.4) staging classification. Staging is very important as treatment depends on the stage. A higher stage has a worse prognosis, and the presence of B symptoms indicates a worse prognosis independent of stage. Clinical staging is carried out with a CT scan of the thorax and abdomen, chest X-ray and, where indicated, bone marrow aspirate and trephine. Most people now feel that pathological staging with a diagnostic laparotomy and splenectomy is not warranted.

Treatment

There are two effective treatments for Hodgkin's disease: radiotherapy and combination chemotherapy. Radiotherapy is curative if all the disease is treated with an adequate dose. Stages IA, IB and IIA disease are usually treated with radiotherapy. Chemotherapy, using four or more drugs often including an anthracycline (Table 14.5), is used for disease stages IIB–IV. Failure to achieve a complete response to treatment or relapse soon after chemotherapy are both poor prognostic factors. A subgroup of relapsed patients may benefit from high-dose chemotherapy and PBSC/ABMT as described above. Patients on chemotherapy are at particular risk from neutropenic sepsis, which is fatal if the diagnosis and treatment are delayed; early referral to the treatment centre is therefore vital. In the long term, infertility may be a problem (particularly in men). In patients with Hodgkin's disease there is an increased risk of second malignancy (AML in the early years, solid tumours later), which is probably related to treatment.

Non-Hodgkin's lymphoma

This is a heterogeneous group of conditions. The incidence is rising, it is more common in older age groups and shows a male preponderance. One-third of cases are extranodal, and may involve the skin, the gastrointestinal tract or any other organ.

Hodgkin's disease
MOPP: mustine, Oncovin (vincristine), procarbazine, prednisolone
Chl(L)V or OPP: chlorambucil (Leukeran), vinblastine or Oncovin, procarbazine, prednisolone
ABVD: Adriamycin (doxorubicin), bleomycin, vinblastine, dacarbazine

Non-Hodgkin's lymphoma
C(H)OP: cyclophosphamide, (hydroxydaunorubicin, doxorubicin), Oncovin, prednisolone
PACE, BOM: prednisolone, Adriamycin (doxorubicin), cyclophosphamide, etoposide, bleomycin, Oncovin, methotrexate + folinic acid
ProMACE, MOPP: prednisolone, methotrexate + folinic acid, Adriamycin, cyclophosphamide, etoposide, MOPP (as above)

Table 14.5   Chemotherapy used to treat malignant lymphoma

B cell	T cell
Low grade	**Low grade**
Lymphocytic[1]	Lymphocytic
Lymphoplasmacytoid	Lymphoepithelioid
	Angioimmunoblastic
Centroblastic-centrocytic, follicular[1]	T zone
	Pleomorphic small cell
High grade	**High grade**
Centroblastic[1]	Pleomorphic medium and large cell
Immunoblastic	Immunoblastic
Large cell anaplastic	Large cell anaplastic
Lymphoblastic	Lymphoblastic

[1] Most frequent types.

Table 14.6 Updated Kiel classification of non-Hodgkin's lymphoma (simplified extract)

There is an increased incidence associated with immunosuppression, autoimmune diseases, certain congenital disorders and AIDS.

The histological classification of non-Hodgkin's lymphoma is controversial. The most commonly used classification systems are the Working Formulation, which is based on cell lineage, type and grade and the Kiel classification, based on lineage, tumour morphology and grade (Table 14.6). A new REAL (revised European–American classification of lymphoma) has recently been proposed.

The clinical features are the same as those for Hodgkin's disease, but the disease is often disseminated and involves bone marrow and extralymphatic organs more frequently. There may be a haemolytic anaemia or paraproteinaemia.

Staging is as for Hodgkin's disease. The Ann Arbor classification is usually applied, though not always appropriate.

Treatment

Non-Hodgkin's lymphoma can be divided into two types: low grade and intermediate/high grade. The low-grade type is a relapsing and remitting condition with a median survival of between 7 and 9 years. Most patients present with disseminated disease. In this group, treatment does not improve survival but is used for symptom control, and is usually with alkylating agents, such as chlorambucil. Radiotherapy is very effective for the control of local symptoms. Newer treatments including fludarabine are under investigation, and while they will probably be effective at inducing a remission, it is unlikely that they will have any effect on overall survival. The use of high-dose chemotherapy and PBSC/ABMT rescue is also under investigation. A significant proportion of these low-grade lymphomas subsequently transform into high-grade lymphoma with a very poor prognosis.

One particular subtype of low-grade non-Hodgkin's lymphoma, follicular low-grade non-Hodgkin's lymphoma, is associated with a characteristic cytogenetic abnormality t(14;18) with translocation of the *BCL-2* gene to the region of the immunoglobulin (Ig) heavy chain locus. This results in constitutive expression of the *BCL-2* protein and resistance of the cells to undergoing programmed cell death (apoptosis).

High-grade non-Hodgkin's lymphoma is an aggressive condition which is treated with combination chemotherapy. Over one-third of cases are cured (unlike the low-grade type). Various chemotherapy regimens have been used (Table 14.5); the reference standard is still CHOP. A number of prognostic factors have been determined. These include age, stage, performance status, serum lactate dehydrogenase and involvement of extranodal sites. Patients with a number of adverse prognostic factors or a poor histological subtype are now treated with high-dose chemotherapy and PBSC/ABMT, in view of the very poor survival with conventional chemotherapy.

Other lymphomas

Mycosis fungoides and Sezary syndrome

Mycosis fungoides is a cutaneous T cell non-Hodgkin's lymphoma. It progresses from a non-specific skin lesion to an indurated skin plaque and then larger nodules. Treatment is usually with external beam irradiation or with PUVA (psoralen and ultraviolet light type A). In the latter stages of the disease there is visceral involvement and a leukaemic phase.

Sezary syndrome is a variant of mycosis fungoides with erythroderma (l'homme rouge) and circulating Sezary cells.

Burkitt's lymphoma

Classical endemic Burkitt's lymphoma is a high-grade non-Hodgkin's lymphoma caused by EBV in patients immunosuppressed by chronic malarial infection. It usually occurs in children and classically involves the jaw, gut, ovaries or testes. There is a characteristic cytogenetic abnormality of chromosome 14 with expression of the *c-MYC* oncogene.

αl Heavy chain disease (immunoproliferative small intestinal disease)

This condition is common in the Middle East and South Africa. It presents with fever, diarrhoea, clubbing and weight loss. Stage A is characterized by infiltration of the mucosa of the small intestine by a clonal proliferation of plasmacytic or lymphoplasmacytic cells. Although clonal this is totally reversible with antibiotics. These plasma cells secrete an abnormal α-immunoglobulin heavy chain. Stage B is characterized by the development of a frankly malignant lymphoma.

Enteropathy associated T cell lymphoma

This is a high-grade T cell lymphoma of the gut, seen in patients with gluten-sensitive enteropathy. It has a very poor prognosis, with a median survival of 18 months.

Multiple myeloma

Multiple myeloma is the most common cause of paraproteinaemia, the other main causes being Waldenstrom's macroglobulinaemia, monoclonal gammopathy of uncertain significance and plasma cell leukaemia. There is a clonal proliferation of cells which usually secrete a paraprotein; this shows as an M band on serum electrophoresis. An excess of light chains, either kappa or lambda, may be excreted in the urine as Bence–Jones protein. Production of the paraprotein may result in suppression of normal production of immunoglobulins (i.e. immunoparesis).

This is a disease of older age groups, with a median onset at 60 years. Men are affected slightly more frequently than women. Patients often present with bone pain, particularly backache, due to bony disease. There may be symptoms and signs of bone marrow failure with anaemia, purpura and infections. Renal failure may occur due to light-chain excretion or hypercalcaemia. Hypergammaglobulinaemia may result in hyperviscosity and immunoparesis will result in increased frequency of infection.

The diagnosis is based on demonstrating: the presence of a paraprotein in the serum; the presence of lytic bone lesion; and identifying Bence Jones proteins. Two of these three conditions make the diagnosis very likely. Bone marrow examination will show infiltration by plasma cells.

Treatment

Good general medical management is vitally important. This includes corrections of anaemia, hypercalcaemia, renal failure and treatment of infection and adequate analgesia. The treatment of myeloma is with chemotherapy. Simple chemotherapy with oral melphalan and prednisolone increases median survival to about 30 months. More aggressive treatment with parenteral chemotherapy will further prolong survival. A selected group of young patients may benefit from high-dose chemotherapy and ABMT/PBSC, followed by maintenance interferon. Radiotherapy is very good for pain relief and control of local disease.

Other disorders

Polycythaemia rubra vera

Polycythaemia rubra vera results from the proliferation of erythroid precursors in the bone marrow. It is due to a defect at the stem cell level and there is also an abnormality of leucocytes and platelets. There is a compensatory increase in plasma volume. It usually occurs in the elderly.

The patient presents with non-specific symptoms of tiredness, bruising, angina, gout and itch. There may be hepatosplenomegaly and the patient may look plethoric. The haemoglobin level is above 18 g/dl. Bone marrow examination shows abnormal erythroid and platelet precursors. Both red cell and plasma volumes are increased, as is the leucocyte alkaline phosphatase level.

Treatment is usually with allopurinol, venesection and chemotherapy with busulfan or hydroxyurea. Radioactive phosphorus (^{32}P) is sometimes used. The condition may progress to myelofibrosis or AML.

Myelofibrosis

Myelofibrosis may arise as a result of polycythaemia rubra vera or *de novo*. There is fibrosis of the bone marrow and extramedullary haemopoiesis. Patients present with massive splenomegaly, anaemia, fever, thrombocytopenia and a raised white cell count. Bone marrow aspirate is 'dry'. Management is essentially supportive, with blood transfusion and splenectomy. The condition may progress to AML.

Waldenstrom's macroglobulinaemia

This is a more benign condition than myeloma and is characterized by clonal lymphocytic infiltration of the bone marrow, production of an IgM paraprotein and the absence of bone lesions. There may be symptoms or signs of hyperviscosity due to the size of the IgM molecule. Treatment is usually with oral alkylating agents; plasmapheresis may be required for hyperviscosity.

Heavy chain disease

In this group of conditions there is secretion of a clonal Ig heavy chain by a lymphoplasmacytic neoplasm. The heavy chain can be α, μ or γ. α1 Heavy chain disease has been discussed above. Y heavy chain disease is a variant of non-Hodgkin's lymphoma. Most patients with μ heavy chain disease have a clinical picture similar to CLL.

Hairy cell leukaemia

This is a rare condition. The cell of origin is unknown. The leukaemic cells have characteristic peanut-shaped nuclei and cytoplasmic projections. Treatment is with splenectomy and/or α-IFN. Recent trials with the new purine analogue 2′-deoxycoformycin have shown response rates of up to 80%.

15

Childhood tumours

R E COLEMAN

Cancer in children is relatively rare, affecting 1 in 600 children before the age of 15 years, but is one of the most common causes of death in childhood. Each year in the UK there are about 1300 new cases of childhood cancer, with an annual incidence rate of about 10 per 100 000 children. Childhood cancer is slightly more common in boys than in girls (1.3:1 M:F ratio).

There are many different types of cancer in children, but approximately one-third will have leukaemia, one-third brain tumours and the final third will have a variety of tumours including Wilms' tumour, neuroblastoma, lymphomas and soft tissue sarcomas (Figure 15.1). In general, paediatric tumours tend to be poorly differentiated, fast growing, very malignant, highly vascular and show early and widespread metastasis.

Particular problems for managing children include those of psycho-social and communication issues, such as providing reassurance, establishing a rapport and explaining treatments. Very young children may need to be sedated or even anaesthetized for certain investigations and treatments. Simple infections, such as measles, mumps or chickenpox, can be fatal in the immunosuppressed child. Metabolic upset such as dangerous dehydration can also occur very rapidly in children. In addition, because of the rarity of childhood cancer, all patients are treated in a

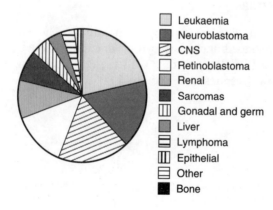

Leukaemia
Neuroblastoma
CNS
Retinoblastoma
Renal
Sarcomas
Gonadal and germ
Liver
Lymphoma
Epithelial
Other
Bone

Figure 15.1 Childhood cancers by type.

few specialized centres around the country and this makes it difficult to maintain family contact.

The causes of childhood cancer are an area of considerable research, as genetic factors play an important part. Indeed, retinoblastoma is the best example of a genetically determined malignancy and Down's syndrome confers a 10–20-fold risk of developing acute leukaemia. Most other childhood tumours do not have a clearly defined inheritance, although the incidence of cancer in siblings is approximately double that of the general population. While in identical twins the incidence, particularly of leukaemia, may be much higher.

Certain other associations of cancer within families have recently become apparent. These include the Li–Fraumeni syndrome characterized by rhabdomyosarcomas and adrenal tumours in the children and breast cancer in the mothers. Other aetiological factors are poorly characterized, although clearly irradiation of the pregnant mother increases the incidence of acute leukaemia in the offspring. Paternal irradiation may also be relevant; a recent study has shown an increased rate of leukaemia among children born to fathers who worked at the Sellafield Nuclear Reprocessing Plant and who had received doses of external ionizing radiation greater than 100 mSv. Paternal smoking may also be relevant, through genetic damage to the development of the sperm.

The outlook for children with cancer has improved dramatically since the introduction of combination chemotherapy. Now at least half of childhood cancers are cured and for many types, survival rates are much higher (Figure 15.2). The best example is ALL where 5-year survival increased by 7-fold from the early 1960s to the early 1980s and continues to improve, as treatments are refined. Considerable

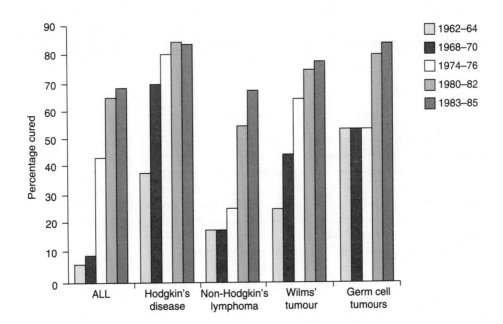

Figure 15.2   Childhood cancer: improvements in survival.

numbers of childhood cancer patients are now surviving into adulthood and many are now having their own children.

Diagnosis of cancer in childhood depends on a high index of suspicion, despite the rarity of cancer in the general population, a careful history and clinical examination, and biopsy of any persistent mass or tissue abnormality for which no cause can be found. Sometimes specific tests are of value, for example, AFP and β-HCG in germ cell tumours and catecholamine excretion for neuroblastoma.

Childhood cancers should only be treated by specialist paediatric oncologists. Many patients will be treated within the context of a national/international clinical trial in an effort to ensure that progress continues and survival prospects improve.

Once the diagnosis is known, assessment and staging investigations should proceed in a planned manner, preferably during the same anaesthetic. If intensive chemotherapy is necessary, a Hickman-style intravenous catheter can be inserted at the same time, through which blood samples can be taken and all drugs administered.

Leukaemia

Childhood leukaemia is most frequently of the ALL type. Chronic and acute myeloid leukaemias account for less than 5% of childhood leukaemia.

ALL is rare at birth, but the incidence increases sharply to a peak at about 4 years of age. The aetiology is unknown, although environmental (irradiation, chemicals), viral (animal experiments, clustering of cases) and genetic (twin studies, associated genetic studies, chromosomal studies) factors have all been implicated. Lymphoblastic leukaemia is characterized by the presence of large immature lymphoblasts throughout the reticuloendothelial system. Their immunocytochemical staining distinguishes them from other white cells, including myeloblasts, and also allows subclassification according to the type of lymphoid cell which has become neoplastic.

Symptoms and signs

Children generally present with the effects of bone marrow infiltration. This may cause anaemia, thrombocytopenia with purpura and haemorrhage, and neutropenia with an increased risk of infection. Other tissues commonly involved include lymph nodes, liver and spleen, all of which can be enlarged. In addition, the child may be lethargic, have a sore throat, appear pale or feverish and may have lost weight. Joint, bone and abdominal pains are sometimes seen. One variant of lymphatic leukaemia is the so-called Sternberg type where the initial presentation is of a large mediastinal mass; leukaemic T cells are subsequently found.

Diagnosis

The differential diagnosis includes infectious mononucleosis, various juvenile collagen-vascular disorders (rheumatic fever, rheumatoid arthritis, systemic lupus erythematosus) and other childhood malignancies. Other causes of pancytopenia must also be considered including aplastic anaemia.

The diagnosis is not normally difficult because leukaemic cells can be found on peripheral blood examination. Occasionally, however, the white blood cell count is normal and only a few abnormal cells can be seen, the so-called 'aleukaemic' leukaemia. Leukaemia must always be confirmed by a bone-marrow examination with appropriate cytology and immunological typing of the leukaemic lymphocyte population involved. Three-quarters of cases are of the so-called 'common' type recognized by the presence of the common ALL antigen (CALLA); less common are T cell ALL (15%), null ALL (8%) and B cell ALL, which is very rare accounting for only about 2% of cases.

The prognosis of the patient may be assessed by a combination of clinical and laboratory indices. The most important are the subtype (with common ALL having a good prognosis and B cell ALL the worst) and the total white blood cell count. A total count of more than $20\ 000 \times 10^9/l$ is associated with a poor prognosis. The prognosis is also better for girls, children aged between 2 and 8 years and those with no significant organomegaly or mediastinal mass.

Treatment

The treatment of ALL has seen major advances over the past 30 years. Treatment can be divided into three phases: induction, consolidation and maintenance. The whole treatment programme may take up to 2 years and throughout this period, intensive medical support is necessary for the patient with blood products, antibiotics and psycho-social support for the patient and family.

For the induction phase, the principle of management is to reduce the population of malignant cells to as near zero as possible by intensive chemotherapy, using a combination of prednisolone, vincristine and asparaginase, usually with either doxorubicin or daunorubicin. Induction therapy usually continues for about 8 weeks after which 90% of patients will be in remission.

Once remission is induced, consolidation is required. This includes prophylactic treatment to the CNS using radiotherapy to the whole brain and intrathecal injections of methotrexate. In addition, high-dose combination chemotherapy may also be required. At the end of this phase, maintenance treatment is given with methotrexate and mercaptopurine. ALL is probably the only malignant disease in which maintenance chemotherapy is still recommended.

For many years it has been realized that despite the excellent initial responses to combination chemotherapy, certain pharmacological 'sanctuary' sites are commonly the site of relapse. The CNS (particularly the meninges) is the most important and hence the reason for routine prophylactic treatment with cranial irradiation and intrathecal chemotherapy. In addition, it is now realized that 10% of boys will develop testicular disease, posing the controversial question of prophylactic testicular irradiation, which results in infertility and reduced testosterone production.

High-dose chemotherapy with autologous bone marrow transplantation and more recently peripheral blood stem cell (PBSC) support is frequently being included in the initial management of patients with a poor prognosis and as salvage therapy for those developing bone marrow relapse after initial induction therapy. Where possible, treatment is given in the context of the Medical Research Council United Kingdom Acute Lymphatic Leukaemia (UKALL) trials which are steadily refining and improving the results of treatment.

Supportive treatment is of vital importance, particularly in the induction phase of treatment. Allopurinol should be given to prevent uric acid nephropathy. In the first few days of treatment, intravenous hydration may be necessary to reduce the chance of the 'tumour lysis syndrome' where potassium and phosphate as well as uric acid may reach dangerously high levels as huge numbers of leukaemic cells break down in response to the chemotherapy.

The prognosis of ALL has improved from it being an invariably fatal disease in the 1950s, with most patients dying within a year of presentation, to being potentially curable with a long-term disease-free survival and a probable cure rate in excess of 70%.

CNS tumours

Neural tumours are the most common paediatric solid tumours. In the CNS the majority of childhood tumours tend to be infratentorial, whereas in the adult most are supratentorial. The group includes astrocytomas, usually cerebellar, medulloblastoma, ependymoma and other gliomas. Surgery is usually the treatment of choice, often followed by CNS irradiation. Chemotherapy is an important component of treatment in medulloblastoma particularly, but also in very young patients with glioma, multi-agent chemotherapy is included in the treatment programme. The overall 5-year survival is about 50%. Unfortunately, some of these survivors have residual CNS defects. A full discussion of CNS tumours is given in Chapter 16 while neuroblastoma and retinoblastoma are discussed below.

Neuroblastoma

Neuroblastoma is a tumour of young children with 50% occurring before the age of 2 years and most occurring below the age of 5 years. The tumour may even be present at birth. It is the most common extracranial tumour of childhood and occurs in 9 out of every million children.

The tumour arises from sympathetic nervous tissue, particularly in the adrenal medulla but also in the neck, mediastinum and pelvis. There is an association with von Recklinghausen's disease but most cases have no recognizable causal factor. Specific chromosome abnormalities are usually seen with deletion of a portion of chromosome 1.

Three histological variants are described. Neuroblastoma which is highly malignant, ganglioneuroma which is a benign encapsulated tumour and ganglioneuroblastoma which is midway between the first two in degree of malignancy. Histologically, the tumour is characterized by densely staining small round cells in neurofibrillary tissue. The cells may group together in an appearance described as rosettes.

The tumour invades locally and also produces lymph-node metastases and disseminates via the bloodstream to the bone marrow and liver. Lung metastases are unusual. Spontaneous maturation and regression may occur, particularly in the newborn and young infant. Interestingly, a much higher incidence of asymptomatic tumours is found in stillborn babies or infants dying from unrelated causes than is seen in the general population.

Symptoms and signs

Symptoms and signs depend on the site of the disease and age at presentation. Abdominal tumours are the most common, and typically present as a distended abdomen due to a large primary tumour mass. Alternatively, a dumb-bell tumour may be seen on the chest X-ray, sometimes with a component within the spinal cord producing spinal compression, Horner's syndrome, cerebellar ataxia and eye-movement disorders. Occasionally, symptoms and signs result from the biological activity of these tumours. Neuroblastomas produce catecholamines, such as adrenaline, noradrenaline and dopamine and the breakdown products vanillylmandelic acid. These substances may cause hypertension, tachycardia, dilated pupils, flushing and diarrhoea.

Investigations

Careful staging of the patient is important and should include a chest X-ray, intravenous pyelogram, skeletal survey and bone-marrow biopsy in all patients. Extensive bone-marrow disease may cause pancytopenia and there may also be obstructive renal impairment with large abdominal masses. Twenty-four hour urine collections should be made to measure catecholamine excretion. The serum ferritin level is also worth measuring as a prognostic factor. Where possible it is also useful to perform an MIBG scan. MIGB (meta-iodobenzylguanidine) is a catecholamine precursor taken up by many of the cells in neuroblastoma, which can be used as a tracer for monitoring progress and also has therapeutic uses for giving targeted irradiation.

Management

If the disease is localized and the tumour can be removed, survival is very good, although such cases are uncommon. Post-operative radiotherapy is given for older children (more than 1 year) or those with poorly differentiated tumours after radical surgical excision. Relatively small doses are usually adequate, thereby reducing the long-term complications of treatment. Another important group of patients are those under the age of 1 year classified as having stage 4S disease by virtue of liver, bone marrow or skin disease. They often remit spontaneously, although gentle chemotherapy or low-dose irradiation may be indicated for pressure symptoms caused by the tumour mass.

Treatment for stage III and IV disease is difficult, relying on combination chemotherapy; cisplatin or carboplatin, etoposide and cyclophosphamide are the most important agents. Intensive chemotherapy using high-dose melphalan and PBSC support improves the prognosis. In addition, therapeutic MIBG treatment may also be used.

Prognosis

The prognosis for localized neuroblastoma is good. More than 90% of patients with stage I and 80% of those with stage II disease are cured. Stage IV disease also has a good prognosis due to the frequency of spontaneous regression. In contrast, patients with true metastatic disease have a very poor prognosis.

Nephroblastoma (Wilms' tumour)

Wilms' tumour of the kidney occurs in 1 in 20 000 children, affecting both sexes equally. The peak age incidence is 3 years with the majority occurring before the age of 5 years. Wilms' tumour is associated with certain rare congenital abnormalities, both of the urogenital tract and elsewhere including aniridia. Occasionally, the tumour is familial and deletions on the short arm of chromosome 11 appear to be important in the development of the tumour.

The tumour arises in the kidney with 5% of cases occurring bilaterally. The tumour usually appears encapsulated with areas of haemorrhage, necrosis and cyst formation within it. Histologically, the tumour is very variable with areas of differentiation into fat, muscle or cartilage associated with embryonal glomerular and renal tubular elements.

The tumour invades locally into the kidney and renal vein. Lymph node metastases are rare with metastatic spread usually occurring via the bloodstream to the lungs.

The tumour typically presents as an intra-abdominal mass in a young child. This is often asymptomatic but may cause pain. Haematuria is sometimes seen and unexplained fever, hypertension, anaemia and weight loss occasionally occur.

Investigation

The extent of the primary tumour should be determined by a CT scan of the abdomen and either abdominal ultrasound or intravenous pyelography. In addition, a full blood count, routine biochemistry, urine analysis and a chest X-ray should be performed before commencing treatment. The tumour is staged according to its extension beyond the renal capsule, the degree of excision and the presence of metastases.

Management

Surgical resection of the tumour is the primary modality. At the time of nephrectomy a regional lymph node dissection should be performed and the contralateral kidney carefully inspected for the presence of a second tumour. Post-operatively, radiotherapy or chemotherapy is given according to the stage of the disease. Those with complete excision of disease retained within the capsule receive a short course of weekly vincristine injections. More extensive tumours are treated with radio-therapy to the renal bed plus combination chemotherapy, while those with stage IV metastatic disease are treated with intensive chemotherapy followed by radio-therapy to the renal bed in those that respond well.

Radiotherapy to the renal bed results in growth retardation of the lumbar vertebrae. The entire width of the vertebral body should be included to avoid scoliotic deformity from differential growth across the vertebral body.

Modern multi-modality treatment has greatly improved the prognosis of this disease. Of those with stage I/II disease 80–90% are cured and even for those with widespread disease a cure rate of 50% is possible.

Retinoblastoma

Retinoblastomas occur almost exclusively in children under the age of 5 years and are bilateral in 30% of cases. It is a rare tumour, present in about 1 in 20 000. The disease follows an autosomal dominant pattern of inheritance, although some patients have no preceding family history. The specific gene location has been identified as the retinoblastoma gene on the long arm of chromosome 13. The tumour typically presents as a white pupil or cat's eye as the tumour reflects incident light. Visual disturbance, strabismus and local pain may be present. Glaucoma may also develop. Metastasis occurs late and is a relatively rare finding.

Management

The treatment depends on the size of the tumour and the state of the other eye. Small tumours may be treatable by laser coagulation and larger tumours are treated with radiotherapy. Radiotherapy can either be given by external beam irradiation or alternatively in the form of a radioactive disc placed over the tumour, which is then removed after an appropriate dose has been administered. Enucleation is avoided where possible but will be necessary if the optic nerve is invaded. Chemotherapy may also be required. The aim of treatment is not only to cure the disease but to preserve as much vision as possible. The prognosis is generally very good.

Histiocytosis

Histiocytosis X is a disease of unknown aetiology characterized by the development of granulomatous lesions with abnormal proliferation of histiocytes. It is commonly believed to be a neoplastic disorder. Three distinct forms are recognized with the clinical course ranging from benign to highly malignant.

Letterer–Siwe disease represents the aggressive end of the spectrum. It presents as an acute disseminated form of the disorder in children below the age of 3 years.

Hepatosplenomegaly, lymphadenopathy, skin, lung and bone infiltrations are found. The disease is usually rapidly fatal despite combination chemotherapy.

In contrast, Hand–Schuller–Christian disease is a chronic disorder occurring at any age but typically in the age group 3–5 years. Lesions are seen in bone and visceral tissues (skin, lung, lymph nodes and liver). The classical triad of cranial lesion, diabetes and exophthalmos is seen in only a small proportion of cases. The course of the disease is slow and may be modified by combination chemotherapy, such as vincristine, doxorubicin and actinomycin D and cyclophosphamide. Patients may survive for many years, although most ultimately succumb, usually from intra-cranial disease and infection.

Eosinophilic granuloma is the least aggressive form of this disease usually pre-senting as solitary lytic bone lesions affecting children aged 5–10 years. The prognosis is usually excellent. Many of the lesions regress spontaneously and if symptomatic respond well to radiotherapy. If and when the disease does become widespread, particularly when clinical deterioration is rapid, chemotherapy can pro-duce useful remissions.

Soft tissue and bone sarcomas

These tumours are largely discussed in Chapter 17. However the most common soft tissue tumour to occur in children is embryonal rhabdosarcoma which differs from the adult alveolar and pleomorphic forms of this disease.

Rhabdosarcoma usually occurs in the first 5 years of life with an incidence of three per million children. They can arise at any site but are most common in the head and neck region particularly around the eye and in the genito-urinary tract. The tumours appear as pink fleshy masses which have been likened to a bunch of grapes (sarcoma botryoides). Microscopically, small darkly staining round cells are seen which are rich in glycogen and contain myofibrils. The disease progresses rapidly with haematogenous spread, particularly to the lungs. In addition, lymph node metastases may occur.

The presenting symptoms depend on the site of origin. Most tumours present as a painless mass. However, nasal obstruction, epistaxis from the nasopharynx, haematuria from the bladder, visual disturbance from the orbit and vaginal bleeding from the vagina or uterus may represent local disease at these sites.

Management

The disease should be staged with routine blood tests, chest X-ray, CT scan of the primary tumour and chest. A bone-marrow examination should be performed as metastases to the bone marrow are quite frequent. The treatment is based on the extent of the tumour and the presence of metastases. However, all cases now receive combination chemotherapy followed by definitive local therapy with surgery or radiotherapy and then further chemotherapy to consolidate the response. For large inoperable tumours or those with metastases, aggressive multi-agent chemotherapy regimens are now being given, sometimes at very high doses requiring PBSC support.

Tumours which are confined to the site of origin have a good prognosis with cure rates of 80%. However, those with metastases do less well with fewer than 20% cured. The best prognosis is seen with tumours of the orbit, bladder, paratesticular region and vagina while those developing in parameningeal sites, prostate or the perineum have a poor prognosis.

Lymphoma

Both Hodgkin's disease and non-Hodgkin's lymphoma may occur in children. These diseases are discussed in full in Chapter 14. Particular features in children include a tendency for non-Hodgkin's lymphoma to be of a very high grade with either diffuse lymphoblastic histology or T cell origin associated with a mediastinal mass. Indeed low-grade non-Hodgkin's lymphoma is very rare in children. Hodgkin's disease tends to be of a subtype with better prognosis and because of the effects of radiotherapy on growth and other organs, chemotherapy is generally preferred.

Germ cell tumours

These are discussed in full in Chapters 11 and 12. In children, the majority are benign but around 20% will be malignant. The distribution of germ cell tumours in children differs from that in adults. The common sites including the ovary, sacrococcygeal region and the mediastinum, retroperitoneum and brain. Treatment is generally with combination chemotherapy and as with adult germ cell tumours the prognosis is good.

In general, the outlook for the child with cancer is now very good. For most types of childhood malignancy it is likely that the child will do well. For a few cancers, survival is still low and more effective treatments need to be found. It is important that all children receive optimum treatment and this is best given in a specialist centre. Improvements in staging and understanding of prognostic factors will ensure that very intensive treatment is only given to those who need it, while less intensive treatments with fewer side-effects can be given to those with a good prognosis. This should result in fewer acute and long-term side-effects and better utilization of precious health-care resources.

There is increasing concern about long-term morbidity from both chemotherapy and radiotherapy. Because of this, patients should continue follow-up well into adulthood and probably for life. Cardiomyopathy, growth and intellectual impairment, infertility and an increased risk of second primary tumours are some of the important late effects of treatment. Although fertility is reduced, especially in girls who have received abdominal irradiation, the risk of cancer and congenital malformations in the children of survivors is similar to that in the general population. In recent years, the importance of counselling and support for the patient and family has been more widely recognized and services have been developed to provide this, including special schooling programmes.

16

Tumours of the CNS

S RAMAKRISHNAN and J D BRADSHAW

Primary tumours of the CNS are uncommon, accounting for less than 2% of all tumours. They can arise at any age, with two age peaks, one in childhood (3–12 years) and the other in later life (50–70 years). CNS tumours are the most common group of solid tumours in childhood, accounting for about 20% of all paediatric neoplasms. Approximately two-thirds of childhood CNS tumours are infratentorial in origin and a similar proportion of tumours in adults are supratentorial. Overall, there is no difference in the sex incidence but astrocytomas are more common in men and meningiomas in women.

There are no known aetiological factors for these tumours. Trauma, chemicals and viruses have been cited, but their role is not established. Some CNS tumours are associated with conditions which have a genetic predisposition. Cerebral lymphomas have been associated with immunosuppression.

Pathology

Malignant tumours of the CNS are unique in that they seldom metastasize outside their system of origin. They are, however, locally invasive and some have a strong tendency to spread along the CSF pathways (e.g. medulloblastoma and dysgerminoma). Different areas in a tumour may show different grades of malignancy, especially in the gliomas, and then the tumour is graded according to the least differentiated tissue present. The degree of malignancy may also increase with time, some tumours gradually becoming more anaplastic. Tumours that are histologically benign can cause pressure symptoms on vital structures within the brain and produce clinical sequelae similar to malignant tumours.

CNS tumours can be classified according to the tissue of origin:

- tumours of neuroglial origin (connective tissue of CNS)
- tumours of the meninges and nerve sheaths
- tumours of embryonal origin
- tumours of the pituitary gland
- other intracranial tumours
- metastatic tumours
- tumours of the spinal cord.

Gliomas

Gliomas comprise approximately 50–60% of all primary CNS tumours.

Astrocytomas

Astrocytomas account for most (about 75%) gliomas. They are graded histo-logically from grade 1 to grade 4 (Kernohan grading system), taking into account features such as mitoses, nuclear atypia, cellularity, vascular endothelial prolifera-tion and necrosis. The better differentiated tumours (grades 1 and 2) are slow growing as opposed to the anaplastic or malignant variants (grades 3 and 4). The term 'glioblastoma multiforme' refers to a rapidly growing malignant tumour which causes extensive haemorrhage, necrosis and considerable distortion of the brain and accounts for more than 75% of all high-grade gliomas in adults. All gliomas, whether benign or malignant, have the tendency to infiltrate the adjacent brain tissue and are usually not well demarcated or encapsulated. Astrocytomas can ex-hibit cystic change.

Oligodendrogliomas

Oligodendrogliomas are tumours arising from oligodendrocytes and account for about 5% of all gliomas. They usually occur in adults and are associated with slow growth but may become anaplastic after many years. They commonly exhibit num-erous foci of calcification, demonstrable radiologically and on histology.

Ependymomas

Ependymomas are tumours arising from the lining of the ventricles. They can also occur in the spinal cord and cauda equina. Approximately 50% are of low-grade malignancy but can cause obstructive symptoms. Anaplastic ependymomas are more common in children and can spread along the CSF pathway. Tumour cells are characteristically oriented around blood vessels.

Medulloblastoma

Medulloblastoma is thought to result from aberrant embryogenesis and arises in the cerebellum from the floor of the fourth ventricle. It usually occurs in the first decade of life, constituting approximately 20% of childhood brain tumours, and is more common in boys. Medulloblastoma occasionally occurs in adults. It is a poorly differentiated, rapidly growing tumour associated with CSF seeding.

Tumours of the meninges and nerve sheaths

These tumours account for about 30% of all primary CNS tumours.

Meningiomas

Meningiomas are solid lobulated tumours arising from the arachnoid layer of the meninges. They are usually well defined or encapsulated and firmly attached by a broad base to the dura mater. The common sites of presentation are the parasagittal region, the sphenoidal wing, the olfactory groove and the convexity of the skull. The majority are benign. Some meningiomas infiltrate the overlying bone and an aggressive variant (malignant meningioma) has been described. Microscopically, meningiomas have a characteristic whorled appearance with areas of calcification and psammoma bodies.

Tumours of the nerve sheaths are believed to originate from Schwann cells and are called **schwannomas** (neurilemmomas). The most common site is the auditory nerve and the tumour is called an **acoustic neuroma**. These are usually slow-growing tumours arising in the cerebellopontine angle and producing unilateral deafness.

Tumours of embryonal origin

Craniopharyngioma

Craniopharyngioma is a tumour which arises from the embryological remnant of Rathke's pouch. It usually develops in children, but may present in early adult life. The tumour typically consists mainly of a cyst cavity, the wall of which contains active cells, sometimes concentrated as a solid tumour. They are usually of low-grade malignancy but can behave aggressively because of their location and invasive potential. They usually develop in the suprasellar region of the brain and can compromise the visual pathways and hypothalamus, resulting in visual failure, diabetes insipidus and hypogonadism.

Chordoma

Chordoma arises from the primitive notochord. It can develop in the caudal (sacrum) or cranial (clivus) ends of the neuraxis. They are histologically benign but have the potential to invade locally especially in bone.

Tumours of the pituitary gland

Pituitary tumours used to be classified as chromophobe, eosinophilic and basophilic adenomas. Chromophobe adenomas are non-functional and produce clinical effects by pressure on the surrounding structures. Eosinophilic tumours secrete growth hormone resulting in acromegaly. Basophilic adenomas secrete adrenocorticotrophic hormone resulting in Cushing's syndrome. The above classification represents the dominant hormonal effect and it is now known that pituitary tumours are capable of producing a range of hormones. In addition to the above, prolactin secreting micro- and macro-adenomas can also occur.

Other intracranial tumours

Tumours of the pineal region include pineal astrocytoma, teratoma, dysgerminoma and pineoblastoma. The last two are often malignant with a tendency for local and CSF pathway spread.

Vascular tumours include haemangioma, haemangioblastoma and arteriovenous malformations.

Primary CNS lymphoma is thought to be of lymphoreticular origin. It occurs more frequently in patients who have received immunosuppressive therapy. It is a highly malignant tumour which invades locally and causes subarachnoid seeding.

Metastatic tumours

Metastatic tumours are very common in the brain and account for approximately 20% of intracranial tumours. They are usually multiple but may be solitary. Common primary sites include lung, breast, kidney, colon, melanoma and lymphoma.

Tumours of the spinal cord

Spinal cord tumours may develop in the extradural or intradural compartments.

Extradural tumours are usually of metastatic origin apart from spinal chordoma. Non-Hodgkin's lymphoma, plasmacytoma and myeloma can also arise in the extradural compartment.

Intradural extramedullary tumours include neurofibroma and meningioma. Neurofibromas are usually attached to nerve roots and are primarily unilateral. They are usually benign and encapsulated. In neurofibromatoses, multiple spinal neurofibromas may occur. Meningiomas may occur anywhere in the intradural compartment.

Intradural intramedullary tumours include astrocytomas, ependymomas and vascular malformations.

Clinical features

The symptoms and signs of CNS tumours may be general or local.

General effects

General effects are related to raised intracranial pressure and result in a classical triad of headache, vomiting and papilloedema. These features may occur individually or in combination and may progress to impairment of mental function, drowsiness, irritability, reduced level of consciousness and coma. The headache is often worse early in the morning and improves during the day. Papilloedema can cause reduced visual acuity and, if prolonged, can result in optic atrophy.

A rise in intracranial pressure can lead to impaction of the brain stem in the opening of the tentorium or of the medulla in the foramen magnum, and either situation can result in rapid death from depression of the vital centres. False localizing signs such as 6th cranial nerve palsy can also occur with raised intracranial pressure. Sudden changes in the level of consciousness or the neurological status may be due to haemorrhage in or around a tumour.

Local effects

Localizing symptoms and signs are directly related to the site of the tumour and result from pressure on, or destruction of, nerve cells and fibres. For example, compression of the optic chiasma by pituitary tumours can result in visual field defects. Frontal lobe tumours can result in personality change and impairment of intellect. Nystagmus and incoordination occur with cerebellar tumours. Damage to the long tract fibres can result in paralysis or sensory disturbances. Tumours of the dominant temporal lobes can result in speech defects. Tumours in the cerebral motor cortex can cause seizures of Jacksonian type or generalized epileptiform fits. Occipital lobe tumours may be associated with visual field defects.

Primary tumours of the spinal cord usually present with pain and loss of neurological function at and below the cord lesion. Depending on the level and extent of the lesion, the patient usually develops motor and/or sensory signs with or without sphincter disturbance. Unilateral intramedullary tumours can result in the Brown–Sequard syndrome where there is loss of pain and temperature sensation below the lesion on the opposite side of the body with weakness and loss of vibration and joint sense below the lesion on the same side of the body. Malignant spinal cord compression is an oncological emergency occurring in approximately 5% of patients with malignancy. It may have an insidious or acute onset with back pain, weakness, loss of sensation and interference with bladder and bowel control. Malignant spinal cord compression can occur at any level but is more common in the thoracic spine. Multiple levels of compression can also occur. Complete paraplegia rapidly develops unless the spinal cord compression is detected and treated early.

Diagnosis and investigations

A full and detailed history and a meticulous clinical examination will usually indicate accurately the site of a tumour in the CNS and sometimes its probable nature. However, a decision about the best form of management requires a very precise knowledge of the extent as well as the site of the lesion, and a firm histological diagnosis.

Plain X-rays of the skull may show evidence of: calcification in a tumour (e.g. craniopharyngioma or oligodendroglioma); erosion of the sella in some pituitary tumours; separation of the cranial sutures secondary to raised intracranial pressure in children; or hyperostosis in meningioma. Tomography and isotope scanning of the brain have been useful in the past in diagnosing brain tumours but have largely been replaced by CT scanning. CT scanning of the brain may show evidence of a space-occupying lesion in the brain. Depending on the nature and extent of the tumour, there may be associated oedema and hydrocephalus. Malignant tumours are usually associated with intravenous contrast enhancement.

Other investigations that may be useful include angiography prior to surgery and MRI. The latter is especially useful for lesions in the spinal cord, brain stem and posterior fossa. Electroencephalography has been used to localize intracranial tumours, but is of limited value. Examination of the CSF is useful in certain clinical situations, for example estimation of tumour markers in pineal dysgerminoma, and cytological examination for the presence of tumour cells in conditions prone to be associated with CSF seeding, such as medulloblastoma, ependymoma and pineoblastoma. For lesions involving the spinal cord, plain radiographs of the spine may show evidence of vertebral collapse or destruction of the pedicles at the level of the compression. Myelography may show evidence of partial or complete obstruction of the spinal canal. An MRI scan of the spine is very useful in determining the level and extent of the spinal cord tumour and is the investigation of choice, if available.

Management

The initial management of intracranial tumours usually involves some form of surgical intervention to establish a histological diagnosis.

Biopsy

Despite accurate modern neuroradiological techniques, it is important to obtain a tissue diagnosis if feasible. This may be simple burr-hole aspiration biopsy or craniotomy with open biopsy. For inaccessible tumours, biopsy using a stereotactic technique is available in most neurosurgical units. A biopsy may not always be conclusive and may only give information on one part of the tumour. It should be used in conjunction with the clinical and radiological features to make a decision on further management. Biopsy can be associated with uncontrollable haemorrhage and post-biopsy oedema.

Debulking surgery

Depending on the size and the location of the tumour, partial resection, attempted total tumour excision or lobectomy may be attempted as an open procedure. Complete surgical removal of intracranial tumours is seldom possible. The microcystic cerebellar childhood astrocytomas and localized grade I cerebral astrocytomas in adults are exceptions. In certain situations, such as in pituitary tumours, subtotal excision using a transnasal trans-sphenoidal approach followed by post-operative radiotherapy would be preferable to attempted radical curative surgical excision, because of possible damage to the visual tracts and development of endocrine dysfunction. Tumours in the brain stem and corpus callosum are unsuitable for debulking surgery because of associated morbidity.

Palliative surgical procedures

These include simple aspiration of cystic tumours to relieve raised intracranial pressure. For recurrent cystic tumours, insertion of an Omaya reservoir allows regular drainage of fluid within the cysts. Insertion of a ventriculoperitoneal shunt is a useful procedure to relieve hydrocephalus.

Role of steroids

High-dose steroid treatment (dexamethasone, 16 mg/day) is a very useful measure in the short-term treatment of raised intracranial pressure prior to definitive treatment with surgery and/or radiotherapy. Long-term use of steroids, however, is associated with significant side-effects.

Role of radiotherapy

The radiosensitivity of CNS tumours varies widely with pineal dysgerminomas being highly radiosensitive and meningiomas and low-grade gliomas being radioresistant. In addition to the sensitivity or resistance of CNS tumour cells, the radiation tolerance of the brain and spinal cord is relevant in deciding the technique, dose, volume and fractionation of radiation therapy. The spinal cord, brain stem and hypothalamus are more sensitive to radiation than the frontal, temporal and occipital lobes, which will tolerate a higher dose of radiation. The radiation dose per fraction is an important factor in CNS radiation tolerance and in view of this, the dose per fraction is usually kept at 2 Gy or less for radical treatment. Age is also relevant, with children under the age of 5 years being more susceptible to the late effects of high-dose radiation.

Radiation therapy with radical intent is usually delivered with the patient's head immobilized with a cellulose acetate head shell for accurate beam directed treatment. The radiation technique, volume, dose and fractionation depend on the nature, location and extent of the tumour. Radiation therapy will produce epilation and in addition, may exacerbate cerebral oedema in the initial phases of treatment.

Role of chemotherapy

Chemotherapy in general has a limited role in the treatment of CNS tumours. The blood–brain barrier has been implicated as a major limiting factor for the entry of systemic cytotoxic agents into the CNS. Chemotherapy, in addition to surgery and radiotherapy, may have a role in certain CNS tumours (e.g. pineal dysgerminoma, cerebral lymphoma, poor prognostic subgroups of medulloblastoma and high-grade gliomas) and clinical studies are investigating this further.

Treatment and prognosis

Low-grade gliomas

Low-grade gliomas should be treated by total or macroscopic excision if feasible. The role of radiotherapy in low-grade gliomas remains controversial. Non-randomized studies suggest significant prolongation in survival with post-operative radiotherapy following incompletely excised low-grade gliomas. However, other authorities feel that radiotherapy does not significantly alter the natural history of the disease. Five-year survival of low-grade gliomas is approximately 50%.

High-grade gliomas

High-grade gliomas are relatively radioresistant. The usual management is surgical debulking (if feasible) followed by post-operative radiotherapy, provided the patient is fit enough to receive treatment. Despite radical doses, cure is unusual and the median survival for glioblastoma multiforme is 8–9 months. Prognostic factors identified for high-grade gliomas are age, performance status, extent of surgery and length of history of seizures.

Medulloblastoma

Initial treatment of medulloblastoma is attempted macroscopic tumour removal. This is usually followed by radical craniospinal radiation to the entire cerebrospinal axis. Adjuvant cytotoxic chemotherapy has been shown to be useful in certain sub-groups of children with poor prognostic features. Treatment of medulloblastoma results in 5-year survival of about 45%.

Meningiomas

Meningiomas are slow-growing tumours and are thought to be radioresistant. Surgery is the treatment of choice. There is some evidence that radiotherapy for incompletely resected or recurrent meningioma may delay disease progression. Acoustic neuromas are also usually managed by surgery, although stereotactic radiotherapy has yielded encouraging results.

Craniopharyngiomas

Surgical treatment is the treatment of choice for craniopharyngiomas. However, it may not be possible to remove the tumour completely and in this situation, post-operative radiation is indicated, especially if there is evidence of residual solid tumour. If the residual disease is predominantly cystic, instillation of ^{90}Y can be carried out. The prognosis is better in children than in adults, with 5-year survival of over 95%.

Pituitary tumours

Pituitary tumours are moderately radiosensitive. However, initial surgery is essential if there is evidence of optic chiasma compression. The development of the transnasal trans-sphenoidal approach to the pituitary fossa has made surgical removal of pituitary tumours much safer. However, complete clearance is virtually impossible and post-operative irradiation is often used. Bromocriptine is also used in reducing elevated levels of prolactin and growth hormone. Studies suggest that more than 75% of patients with acromegaly and 75–80% of patients with chromophobe adenomas are clinically controlled with radiation. Adult patients with Cushing's disease do not do as well with fewer than 50% being controlled with radiation.

Cerebral metastases

The treatment of cerebral metastases is palliative in intent. Management depends on factors such as the age of the patient, performance status, number of metastases, extent of extracranial systemic disease and the underlying primary. High-dose steroids alone may be appropriate therapy in some patients. Occasionally, surgical removal of an apparently solitary metastatic deposit in an accessible site may be indicated, followed by palliative radiotherapy. Palliative radiotherapy to the whole brain may produce symptom relief and prolong survival by a few months.

Primary spinal cord tumours

Primary spinal cord tumours should be treated by surgical excision or debulking. The technical difficulty of achieving total removal of spinal cord tumours makes post-operative radiotherapy necessary in most cases.

Malignant spinal cord compression

Malignant spinal cord compression requires urgent treatment. The optimal management remains controversial. Surgery, radiotherapy and steroids are used singly or in combination. The management has to be individualized and depends on the patient's general condition, performance status, extent and duration of spinal cord compression, nature, extent and prognosis of the primary malignancy and the stability of the spine. Decompressive laminectomy is associated with some morbidity, but may be indicated for patients with good performance status, a short history of paraparesis, and a solitary level of compression in a surgically accessible site, especially in radioresistant tumours such as melanoma and renal cell carcinoma. Radiotherapy is usually palliative and is given either as a primary treatment or post-operatively. The overall prognosis of malignant spinal cord compression remains very poor and is related to the pre-treatment neurological status and the radio-responsiveness of the primary malignancy. Patients with established paraplegia and sphincter involvement are unlikely to improve with surgery or radiotherapy. In such patients, radiotherapy may be indicated for pain control.

17

Soft tissue and bone tumours

M H ROBINSON

Sarcomas are rare and as a result are commonly mismanaged. They may develop in somatic or visceral tissues.

Soft tissue sarcoma in adults

The soft somatic tissues comprise fibrous and adipose tissue, vessels, lymphatics, nerves, smooth and striated muscle, fascia and synovium. They develop from the primitive mesenchyme within the mesoderm with some neuroectodermal contribution and determine the shape of the human body.

Epidemiology and aetiology

Soft tissue sarcomas account for 1% of adult cancers with an incidence of 37 cases per million persons a year. Approximately 1200 new cases are reported each year in the UK. They are relatively more common in children (6–7%) because of the reduced number of sarcomas in this group.

In the majority of cases there is no clear aetiology. However, there are well-established associations with genetically linked disorders, such as von Recklinghausen's neurofibromatosis, tuberous sclerosis, the basal cell naevus and Li–Fraumeni syndromes.

Following a latent period of 5–25 years, a small proportion (<1%) of adults exposed to therapeutic doses of ionizing radiation develop sarcomas. This is more common in children receiving both radiotherapy and chemotherapy (18%).

Patients often give a history of trauma but it is not clear whether this is causative or coincidental.

Dioxin in the form of herbicide or defoliant (Agent Orange) has been implicated as causing an increased incidence of soft tissue sarcoma. However, this association is not proved.

Many soft tissue tumours have consistent chromosome rearrangements. Chromosome translocations are the most common type. For example the translocation t(x;18) (p11.2;q11.2) is specific for synovial sarcoma and seen in about 80% of cases.

Diagnosis

The importance of an experienced pathologist diagnosing sarcoma cannot be overemphasized. Light microscopy alone may be adequate for many sarcomas, but immunochemistry and electron microscopy may be invaluable.

Despite no uniform grading system for soft tissue sarcoma, grade, however determined, is the most important factor determining the risk of metastasis and thus death in all series. It is clear that a universally agreed method of grading should form the basis of any agreed staging system. Assessment of a combination of pleo-morphism, cellularity, mitotic count and necrosis is often used to determine grade. The majority of patients (75–80%) fall into the high-grade category.

Various staging systems have been used in an effort to predict patient outcome and help to select patients with poor prognosis for adjuvant therapy. Tumour grade is an important determinant of stage in all systems. The most commonly used staging system is that of the Union Internationale Contre le Cancer (UICC) which subdivides stages by tumour size, nodal involvement and the presence of metastases at presentation.

Biopsy

A histological diagnosis of a soft tissue lesion must be obtained before treatment is carried out. Because soft tissue sarcomas are rare, the diagnosis is often unsuspected at the time of presentation and an inappropriate biopsy is performed.

Often patients are referred for definitive management after excisional biopsy. This is a common practice which should be avoided as the exact site of the tumour is then impossible to determine by pre-operative imaging. A further operation is usually required as a tumour will be found in 50% of re-excised specimens.

Investigations

Laboratory investigations need not go beyond a full blood count, assessing electro-lyte levels and estimating liver function

The primary site should be evaluated radiologically using either a CT scan or MRI. MRI may provide a better demonstration of the location and extent of the tumour pre-operatively than CT, but it is not clear that this often influences the choice of operation.

Treatment

Where a lesion is likely to be a soft tissue sarcoma the patient should be referred to a surgeon experienced in the multi-disciplinary treatment of these tumours before biopsy is carried out. Soft tissue sarcomas have a high propensity for local recurrence. Much of this is probably related to the inadequate way in which many of them have been managed in the past. They commonly grow to a large size in many sites before presentation and spread along fascial planes. They often have a pseudocapsule and it is common for the unwary surgeon to comment on how easily they appear to 'shell out'. Surgery initially evolved from very local excision to radical ablative surgery with amputation above the proximal joint in 50% of extremity tumours. In recent years, the value of limited surgical resection with post-operative adjuvant high-dose radiotherapy has been confirmed. Results of treatment at other sites less amenable to adequate surgical clearance (e.g. retroperitoneum and head and neck) are less satisfactory. Because of the varied sites where lesions appear, a surgical team handling them must have many varied skills including the ability to reconstruct and to repair.

Radiotherapy

The use of adjuvant radiotherapy either pre-operatively or post-operatively sig-nificantly improves the prospects of local control in most patients. Its precise indications have not been subjected to randomized clinical trials. However, local recurrence is such a common phenomenon following surgery alone that unless a tumour is low grade and resected with a wide and adequate clearance then adjuvant radiotherapy is indicated.

Radiotherapy alone may be used in high doses to palliate inoperable lesions or where concomitant disease precludes appropriate definitive surgery.

Chemotherapy

Chemosensitive tumours

Most adult soft tissue sarcomas are chemoresistant. However, there is a small group of tumours, characterized by the t(11;22) translocation (extraskeletal Ewing's, peripheral neuroectodermal tumours and Askin's tumour) for which chemotherapy is the primary treatment. Routine use of combinations including vincristine, doxorubicin, cyclophosphamide and actinomycin D have transformed the prognosis of localized Ewing's sarcoma from less than 10% at 5 years to 40%. Recently, ifosfamide has been used in place of cyclophosphamide with success. However, patients with metastases on presentation still have a dismal prognosis and the use of high-dose chemotherapy with ABMT or PBSC infusion is being explored.

Chemoresistant sarcomas

Despite considerable research the activity of cytotoxics in adult soft tissue sarcomas remains disappointing. Single agent doxorubicin is the most active agent with reported response rates of 15–35%. There is little evidence that combination therapy produces superior response rates to high doses of single agent doxorubicin on its own and none that it improves survival. The only other potentially valuable first-line drug is ifosfamide.

Prognosis

The overall survival of patients with extremity soft tissue sarcoma is 35–69% depending on patient selection. In general, young age, extremity tumour, small size and low-grade histology are good prognostic factors.

Sarcomas of children

Rhabdomyosarcoma

These form 5% of all solid tumours in children and are the most common tumours in children under 15 years of age. They occur in 4.5 per million whites and 1.3 per million blacks. There is an overall 70% 2-year survival. This is determined by the extent at diagnosis, the primary site and histology.

Epidemiology

Head and neck and genitourinary tumours peak at 2–6 years of age. Trunk and extremity tumours peak at 14–18 years. They are associated with neurofibromatosis, Gorlin's basal cell naevus and fetal alcohol syndrome. There may be an association with an increased incidence of breast cancer in relatives and an increased incidence of rhabdomyosarcoma in the siblings of patients with brain and adrenocortical tumours. Alveolar rhabdomyosarcomas are associated with t(2;13) (q37;q14) chromosome changes.

Pathology

The largest group of tumours occur in the head and neck (35%) and the most common site is the orbit. Of the remainder, 21% are genitourinary, 18% extremity, 7% trunk and 7% retroperitoneal. Forty to sixty per cent are embryonal rhabdomyosarcomas which resemble primitive muscle. Alveolar rhabdomyosarcomas occur in older children, particularly in the extremity and perineal region; they spread to nodes and have a worse prognosis. Pleomorphic rhabdomyosarcoma is seen in adults and is rare.

Presentation

The tumours present in infants with a grape like botryoides variant. In young patients they present in the head and neck or the genitourinary system. In adolescence they present with a painless extremity lesion.

The margins of the primary tumour are often indistinct because of its pseudocapsule and they are difficult to define on physical examination and at operation.

Spread to lymph nodes occurs uncommonly but varies according to site.

Blood-borne spread has occurred in 10–20% by presentation and usually involves the lungs, bone, bone marrow or liver. This is revealed by clinical examination or by the use of CT scanning of the primary site and chest, bone scan and bone marrow. If the primary tumour is in the head and neck then an MRI scan should be performed and CSF examined.

Staging

These tumours are staged according to the involvement of other structures, their size in relation to 5 cm and the presence or absence of metastasis.

Treatment

After a biopsy, orbital, parameningeal, vaginal and prostate tumours are initially treated with chemotherapy followed by radiotherapy. Truncal extremity, paratesticular tumours are treated by surgery and chemotherapy. Radiotherapy is used where there is microscopic residuum following surgery. The cytotoxic drugs most often used are actinomycin D, vincristine and cyclophosphamide.

Bone sarcomas

Malignant tumours arising from the skeletal system represent only 0.2% of all primary cancers. Approximately 550 new cases occur in the UK annually.

Osteosarcoma and Ewing's sarcoma are the two common bone tumours. They occur mainly during childhood and adolescence. Other types (e.g. fibrosarcoma, chondrosarcoma, malignant fibrous histiocytoma and osteogenic sarcoma arising in Paget's disease) that usually develop after skeletal maturity are less common. These are sometimes associated with benign bony tumours caused by previous radiation.

Bone tumours, unlike carcinomas, disseminate almost exclusively through the blood, particularly to the lung.

Most experience has been obtained in the treatment of osteosarcoma. As a result the surgical, chemotherapeutic and radiotherapeutic principles developed in the treatment of osteosarcomas form the basis of the treatment strategy for most of the other high-grade bone sarcomas.

The development of centres with a specific interest in these tumours has been an important factor in the evolution of successful treatment regimens. Limb-sparing surgery has been developed and advances in orthopaedics, bioengineering, radiographic imaging, radiotherapy and chemotherapy have contributed to safer, more reliable surgical procedures. CT and MRI have increased the accuracy of pre-operative evaluation of the local anatomy and increased the probability of safe resection.

Adjuvant chemotherapy has increased overall survival from 15–20% with surgery alone to 55–80%. Pre-operative and post-operative chemotherapy regimens are being evaluated and their effect on the tumour and impact on the choice of operative procedure and survival studied.

Radiotherapy is now less often used in the management of osteosarcoma. It is still indicated where the surgical clearance is inadequate and is helpful in the palliation of metastatic bone lesions.

Osteogenic sarcoma appearing in elderly patients with Paget's disease is rare and not chemosensitive. It has a dismal prognosis.

Ewing's sarcoma

Ewing's sarcoma was first described by James Ewing in 1921 as a bone tumour composed of small round cells occurring in the mid shaft of long bones or flat bones of the trunk. Recent evidence suggests that it is probably derived from primitive neural tissue. Long-term disease-free survival has increased from less than 15% to over 50% in the last 20–30 years.

Ewing's sarcoma occurs most frequently in the second decade of life and is rare before 5 years of age or after 30. Men predominate after the age of 13 and taller individuals are more likely to develop the disease. There is an extremely low incidence of Ewing's sarcoma in the Chinese and in African and American blacks. The incidence in white children under 15 is 1.7 per million per year. It has not been associated with congenital syndromes but has been associated with skeletal abnormalities, such as enchondroma, aneurysmal bone cyst, genitourinary abnormalities like hypospadias and duplication of the renal collecting systems and retinoblastoma.

Chromosomal translocation t(11;22) is characteristic and is the same as that of peripheral neuroepithelioma. This has led to the view that they have a common origin.

Diagnosis

Under the microscope, Ewing's sarcoma appears as an undifferentiated round cell tumour. It is diagnosed by pathologists only after exclusion of other small round blue cell tumours of childhood. These include bone sarcomas, rhabdomyosarcoma, lymphoma, neuroblastoma and peripheral neuroepithelioma. Electron microscopy and immunocytochemistry are essential.

Ewing's sarcoma most commonly presents in the femur and bones of the pelvis but may affect any bone and often originates in the axial skeleton, unlike osteosarcoma. In the first Intergroup Ewing's sarcoma study, 20% appeared in the pelvis and sacrum, 31% in the proximal extremity, 27% in the distal extremity and 14% in other sites (e.g. ribs and vertebrae).

Most patients present with pain and swelling in the affected region. Systemic symptoms such as fatigue, weight loss and fever occur, particularly in those with metastatic disease.

Metastatic disease occurs in 14–50% at presentation, depending on the thoroughness of the staging. Metastasis is predominantly haematogenous, although lymph node involvement may rarely occur. The lung is the most common site.

There is no uniform staging system in Ewing's sarcoma but increasing tumour size is a poor prognostic factor, as is extraosseous extension. The most favourable prognostic factors are distal primary tumour and the absence of metastases at presentation. Pelvic and sacral sites are the least favourable. Response to initial chemotherapy is a strong predictor of long-term local control.

Treatment

Every patient should be treated with curative intent. The use of surgery has become more widespread over recent years. The generally accepted indications for primary resection are a lesion in an expendable bone, such as a rib, clavicle, fibula or individual bones of the feet, or a lesion in the pelvic region. Amputation is indicated for an unmanageable pathological fracture or if the tumour arises at or below the knee in a young child and a major uncorrectable deformity is expected from radiotherapy.

Before the availability of chemotherapy, local control of Ewing's sarcoma was achieved in 40–80% of patients with radiotherapy.

At least three courses of chemotherapy are usually given before radiotherapy in current treatment protocols. Vincristine, actinomycin D, doxorubicin and cyclophosphamide are the most commonly used drugs.

18

Skin cancer

B W HANCOCK and J D BRADSHAW

Skin cancer is one of the most common human malignancies. Basal cell carcinoma accounts for over half, and squamous cell carcinoma for over a quarter, of all skin cancer. The remainder is made up of melanoma, secondary skin metastases, lymphoma and various other uncommon lesions.

Basal cell carcinoma

Basal cell carcinoma (rodent ulcer) occurs with greater incidence in white races with excessive sunlight exposure, as for example in Australia. It may occur in a dominantly inherited condition, the basal cell naevus syndrome. About three-quarters of basal cell carcinomas arise in the head and neck region, characteristically as an ulcerated nodule. Clinically there may be some difficulty in distinguishing the lesion from kerato-acanthoma, which typically has a central core of keratin. The remainder of basal cell carcinomas occur elsewhere on the body; occasional difficulty is experienced in distinguishing them from solar keratoses, though the latter do not have the typical raised rolled edges of the rodent ulcer.

Metastases are very rare from basal cell carcinoma. If death occurs it is usually from infiltration of vital structures, particularly the brain, where infection is often the cause of death.

Treatment

Treatment is curative in over 90% of cases and this can be by surgical excision (if easily accessible) or by local radiotherapy. Other less favoured methods of treatment include electrocautery, cryosurgery and topical cytotoxic chemotherapy (e.g. fluorouracil ointment). In general, the patient can receive out-patient treatment unless very elderly or otherwise infirm. Great care must be taken to ensure a good cosmetic result in facial lesions.

Recurrent lesions can frequently be cured using the form of treatment alternative to that first used.

Squamous cell carcinoma

Squamous cell carcinoma occurs with increased frequency in non-pigmented skin, with excessive sunlight exposure, with chemical carcinogenesis (e.g. with coal tar products), and with chronic irritation. A recessively inherited skin condition, xeroderma pigmentosum, is associated with development of squamous cell carcinoma. Over half of the lesions occur in the head and neck region and about a quarter on the arms and hands.

Bowen's disease usually manifests as brownish–red crusted or eroded skin plaques. It is a form of intraepidermal carcinoma which may become invasive after a period of months or years. It is also acknowledged to be a marker of internal malignancy, particularly bronchial carcinoma.

Differential diagnosis of squamous carcinoma from basal cell carcinoma and from solar keratosis may be difficult. The squamous lesion is frequently nodular and ulcerated, but may be flat and keratotic. Histological confirmation is required. At the same time, an idea of the degree of differentiation and local invasion can be obtained.

Treatment

Localized lesions, which are well differentiated histologically and forming keratin pearls, are curable in more than 90% of cases by adequate excisional surgery, though results with radiotherapy are also excellent. Larger, poorly differentiated lesions may infiltrate extensively and may metastasize by lymphatic and vascular invasion. Surgery may still be appropriate but radiotherapy is particularly useful in this group. Disseminated disease occasionally responds to combination cytotoxic chemotherapy.

Malignant melanoma

Malignant melanoma, a tumour which strikes fear into the heart of even the most experienced of oncologists, is in fact an uncommon tumour, accounting for about 1% of total cancers. In the skin, it is seen with most frequency, as with basal cell and squamous cell lesions, in fair-skinned races exposed to excessive sunlight, as for example in Australia. It is twice as common in women as in men and its incidence and mortality are increasing.

Pathology

Pathologically skin melanoma is divided into three types:

- superficial spreading melanoma, flat and extending, nearly black in colour – the commonest type

- nodular melanoma, sometimes ulcerated and usually dark brown
- lentigo maligna, a flat dark brown lesion occurring classically on the head and neck region of the older patient.

Occasionally a melanoma may not be pigmented (amelanotic melanoma). Survival is best with lentigo maligna and worst with nodular melanoma; superficial spreading melanoma comes between these two.

Prognosis also depends on the level of invasion in the skin of the melanoma. The deeper the spread, the worse the prognosis.

Differential diagnosis

Malignant melanoma developing in a pigmented mole is uncommon, but may occur more frequently in naevi on the palms and soles. A difficult differential diagnostic problem is, of course, between the mole and the malignant melanoma. In general, lesions with changing size or pigmentation, ulceration or bleeding, should be excised and examined histologically.

Treatment

Treatment of the primary melanoma must be by adequate excisional surgery. For shallow localized lesions survival figures are greater than 90% at 5 years. Once metastasis has occurred, the outlook is much worse with 5-year survival less than 30%. Spread occurs via superficial lymphatics, giving satellite lesions, via deep lymphatics to regional lymph nodes and via the bloodstream most often to the lungs, liver and brain. Block dissection of regional nodes or regional arterial perfusion of cytotoxic agents is occasionally effective. In general, radiotherapy and chemotherapy with agents such as dacarbazine and IFN have little to offer except in palliation. Experimental approaches are being explored e.g. biological therapy, see Chapter 6.

Malignant lymphoma

Malignant lymphoma occurs occasionally as true cutaneous deposits, particularly in non-Hodgkin's lymphoma. Specific T cell skin lymphomas are also seen (see Chapter 11). The Sezary syndrome, of erythroderma with lymphocytic skin infiltration and abnormal blood lymphocytes, and mycosis fungoides, a cutaneous lymphoma characteristically progressing from non-specific 'premycotic' erythroderma to a stage of indurated neoplastic plaques, can both develop into systemic lymphoreticular malignancies. Treatment of isolated lymphoma deposits by radiotherapy gives excellent results. The treatment of widespread lymphoma is much less satisfactory. For skin lesions, PUVA therapy is helpful in many patients. Superficial whole-body irradiation with electrons and systemic chemotherapy are other, later options.

Metastatic skin tumours

Metastatic skin tumours, particularly from breast, lung or gastrointestinal tract, are not usually difficult to diagnose. Treatment is palliative and most often by irradiation, particularly when the lesion is ulcerated or painful.

Other rare tumours

Other rare tumours can arise from structures in the dermis, for example from blood vessels, fibrous tissue and sweat glands. Treatment of these is primarily by excisional surgery.

Kaposi's sarcoma

Kaposi's sarcoma probably arises from the skin blood vessels and has a classical histological appearance. Though clinically often a slowly progressive multifocal skin disease, widespread visceral changes occur eventually in the majority of patients. Treatment of the skin lesion is by surgery or radiotherapy. Disseminated disease occasionally responds to chemotherapy. There is an increased incidence of second cancer (particularly of the reticuloendothelial system) in patients with Kaposi's sarcoma. This neoplasm is a common feature in AIDS; its behaviour is much more aggressive in this group.

19

Paraneoplastic and hormonal syndromes associated with tumours

P C LORIGAN and B W HANCOCK

Cancers manifest their presence in three main ways, firstly by the presence of the primary tumour and its local spread, secondly by metastasis to secondary sites, and thirdly by remote non-metastatic (paraneoplastic) effects. The frequency of occurrence of paraneoplastic syndromes is unknown. Some of these remote effects of malignancy may be due to the secretion of hormones appropriate to the tumour's tissue of origin. The aetiology of the other paraneoplastic phenomena is multifactorial and many are poorly understood; possible mechanisms are shown in Table 19.1.

Endocrine manifestations

Many hormones and peptides secreted by tumours have been identified. Some of these have recognized self-stimulatory (autocrine), distant (endocrine) and local effects (paracrine). The function of many is unknown. Table 19.2 shows the tumours which are known to produce endocrine effects. The differential diagnosis of paraneoplastic endocrine effects includes hormone production by benign cells, organ infiltration by tumour, alteration of hormone production by therapy or infection, or multiple endocrine neoplasia.

The most common tumour which frequently produces endocrine effects is small cell lung carcinoma.

1	Release of substances which may have an autocrine, paracrine or endocrine function (e.g. polypeptide hormones, growth factors, peptides, fetal proteins, prostaglandin, immunoglobin, enzymes)
2	Immune response 　　Autoimmune 　　Immune complex
3	Production of a non-functioning blocking hormone or ectopic receptor production
4	Release into the circulation of compounds not usually found there
5	Unknown

Table 19.1 Aetiology and pathogenesis of paraneoplastic syndromes

Tumour	Hormone	Endocrine effect
Small cell lung cancer Non-small cell lung cancer	Adrenocorticotrophic hormone	Cushing's syndrome
Small cell lung cancer	Antidiuretic hormone	Inappropriate antidiuresis
Non-small cell lung cancer	Atrial natriuretic hormone	Inappropriate natriuresis and diuresis
Lung cancer (all types especially squamous cell)	Parathyroid hormone	Non-metastatic hypercalcaemia
Non-small cell lung cancer Small cell lung cancer	Oestrogen	Gynaecomastia
Lung cancer (all types) Choriocarcinoma	Thyroid stimulating hormone	Hyperthyroidism
Medullary carcinoma thyroid Lung cancer (all types)	Calcitonin	No syndrome
Carcinoid	Growth hormone	Acromegaly
Pancreatic carcinoma	Insulin Insulin like growth factor (I and II) Somatomedins	Insulin-like activity

Table 19.2   Endocrine effects of some tumours

Adrenocortical hyperplasia

Adrenocortical hyperplasia as a result of ectopic production of ACTH was the first paraneoplastic endocrine syndrome to be described. The onset of this form of Cushing's syndrome is rapid with biochemical disturbance occurring before the other physical manifestations. The tumour secretes 'big ACTH' which also contains melanocyte stimulating hormone. Patients may present with respiratory symptoms due to the primary tumour, increasing pigmentation (due to melanocyte stimulating hormone), weight loss due to malignancy and the biochemical abnormalities of Cushing's syndrome. It is rare for the patient to have the physical stigmata of Cushing's syndrome.

Hypercalcaemia

Hypercalcaemia is common in cancer patients, occurring in 10% of cases. In the majority of cases, it is caused by bony metastases. Malignant cells metastatic to bone may cause stimulation of osteoclasts and reabsorption of bone, resulting in hypercalcaemia. In 10–15% of cases, hypercalcaemia is due to production by the tumour of parathyroid hormone related peptide (PTHRP). This is similar in structure and function to parathyroid hormone (PTH). The gene for PTHRP is on a different chromosome to that for PTH. It may be secreted in very low amounts in normal individuals while in malignancy it may be secreted in large amounts. A number of other factors may be involved in the hypercalcaemia of malignancy. These include renal function, prostaglandin secretion and thyroid function. Although some tumours produce large quantities of calcitonin, a clinical effect of this has yet to be described.

Hyponatraemia

Hyponatraemia may be the result of the syndrome of inappropriate antidiuretic hormone (SIADH) production, or inappropriate secretion of natriuretic hormone. Both will lead to hyponatraemia. SIADH is most commonly associated with small cell lung cancer, but occurs in a number of other conditions and as a result of treatment with the drug vincristine. Classically the urine is inappropriately concentrated in the face of a dilute serum (i.e. the patient is conserving water inappropriately). Treatment is with fluid restriction, treatment of the underlying cause, and with demeclocycline, which blocks the effect of antidiuretic hormone on the distal tubules. There are many non-paraneoplastic causes for hyponatraemia including dehydration, fluid overload, Addison's disease and general debility.

Hypoglycaemia

Insulinomas may produce insulin. Other tumours, especially retroperitoneal sarcomas, hepatoma and peritoneal mesothelioma, can all produce hypoglycaemia. This may be due to production of insulin-like peptides. It is unlikely to be due to 'massive glucose utilization' or liver infiltration.

Autocrine/paracrine effects

Many growth factors and peptides produced by tumours have been identified. The function of many of them remains unknown, but some of them have been shown to have autocrine and paracrine effects. Autocrine factors for small cell lung cancer have been identified, their receptors characterized and blocking drugs for their receptors developed. These are currently in early clinical trials. Interleukin-6 is an autocrine factor for plasma cells. A receptor blocker would, theoretically, inhibit the growth of myeloma. Alternatively IL-6 can be used to synchronize myeloma cells in cycle, rendering them more susceptible to chemotherapy.

   In general, the paracrine and endocrine effects of malignancy reflect the stage of the underlying disease. Treatment is therefore directed at treating the underlying condition.

Neurological manifestations

Up to 17% of cancer patients have neurological problems. These are usually due to metastatic disease, or fluid, electrolyte or other metabolic abnormalities. Some neurological abnormalities associated with malignancy are true paraneoplastic phenomena. These are usually caused by autoimmune phenomena, with the tumour sharing antigens with normal tissue. Unlike most other paraneoplastic syndromes, which run a course parallel to the malignancy, this is often not the case with neurological paraneoplastic syndromes. Some neurological phenomena occur almost solely as paraneoplastic syndromes (e.g. Eaton–Lambert syndrome).

Cerebrum and cranial nerves

Paraneoplastic syndromes involving the brain and cranial nerves are less common than those affecting other areas of the neuromuscular axis. Subacute cerebellar degeneration is most commonly associated with lung cancer and is characterized by progressive cerebellar failure with ataxia, dysarthria, hypotonia and pendular reflexes. The immunopathogenesis of this condition is now well understood, and diagnostic autoantibodies have been characterized. Dementia is more common in cancer patients than in the normal population, and is often associated with abnormalities in other areas of the CNS. Presentation may be acute or chronic. Optic neuritis due to demyelination and photosensitivity, ring scotomas and visual field loss due to retinal ganglion cell loss have both been described as autoimmune phenomena associated with malignancy.

Spinal cord

Approximately 10% of patients with amyotrophic lateral sclerosis have cancer. The patients have both upper and lower motor neuron disease with spasticity, wasting, extensor plantar reflexes and fasciculations. Subacute motor neuropathy is strongly associated with malignancy; patients have slowly progressing lower motor neuron weakness.

Peripheral nerves

Peripheral nerves are the most common neurological site affected in paraneoplastic syndromes. Pure sensory neuropathy is uncommon, but strongly associated with malignancy. Mixed sensory motor neuropathy is more common. Recovery is rare, even with successful treatment of the underlying malignancy.

Muscle and neuromuscular function

Between 10% and 30% of patients with dermatomyositis and polymyositis have an associated malignancy. These patients have proximal muscle weakness which progresses slowly and is associated with raised serum muscle enzymes and characteristic electromyographic and histological findings.

Eaton–Lambert syndrome

This unusual condition is usually associated with small cell lung carcinoma. The syndrome may pre-date diagnosis by up to 3 years. There is weakness of the muscles of the proximal limbs and pelvis. This weakness improves with exercise. There is a failure of release of acetylcholine from the terminal axons. The Tensilon (edrophonium) test (response to anticholinesterase) is negative. Treatment is with guanidine. Treatment of the underlying malignancy may result in some improvement.

Myasthenia gravis

This is an autoimmune disorder characterized by weakness of the external ocular muscles, cranial nerves and the upper limbs. The weakness worsens with exercise. It is associated with a thyoma in 10–15% of cases. There is acetylcholine receptor deficiency. The Tensilon test is positive.

Haematological manifestations

Abnormalities in all cell lines and in clotting factors have been reported in cancer.

Anaemia

Anaemia may be caused by autoimmune haemolysis, by bleeding, by vitamin deficiencies and by infiltration of the bone marrow by malignant cells. Most commonly there is the normochromic normocytic anaemia of chronic disease, the aetiology of which is uncertain.

Erythrocytosis

Erythrocytosis is most commonly seen in hypernephroma, hepatoma and cerebellar haemangioblastoma, probably due to erythropoietin secretion by these tumours. ACTH, aldosterone, testosterone and catecholamines can also increase the production of red cells.

White cell and platelet abnormalities

Granulocytosis is associated with lung, stomach and pancreatic carcinoma and may be due to production of cytokines by these tumours. Granulocytopenia is associated with thymoma. Lymphopenia is a poor prognostic factor in untreated lymphoma. Thrombocytosis is relatively frequent in many tumours, again probably due to cytokine production. Idiopathic thrombocytopenia occurs in a number of lympho-proliferative disorders.

Coagulation disorders

Migratory thrombophlebitis is usually associated with mucin-producing tumours, but it is also found in association with lung, ovary and prostate cancer. Non-infective thrombotic endocarditis with large friable fibrinous valvular vegetations may also be found.

Disseminated intravascular coagulation

There is an abnormality of clotting in up to 90% of patients with cancer. This may lead to overcompensated intravascular coagulation with consumption of clotting factors. As an acute event this may lead to an acute haemorrhage diathesis. Chronic low-grade DIC tends to be of a thrombotic nature.

Renal lesions

Paraneoplastic phenomena affecting the kidneys are usually immune mediated and give rise to the nephrotic syndrome. Renal involvement by amyloid also occurs.

Skin lesions

Skin lesions associated with malignancy are shown in Table 19.3.

Other manifestations

Hepatopathy

Hepatopathy is deranged liver function, not due to liver involvement by metastatic disease. Hepatopathy occurs in a small percentage of patients.

Anorexia, cachexia and taste disturbance

These are common problems in patients with cancer. They bear no relationship to the site, stage or type of disease. Despite reduced caloric intake, the basal metabolic rate fails to adjust downwards. A number of cytokines have been implicated.

Disorder	Description	Comments
Pigmented		
Acanthosis nigricans	Hyperkeratosis and pigmentation, especially of axillae, neck, flexures and anogenital regions	Usually intra-abdominal malignancy, may be due to excretion of TGF-α
Tripe palms	Exaggerated ridges on palms	Associated with lung and gastric calcium and with acanthosis nigricans
Leser–Trelat	Sudden development of multiple seborrhoeic warts	Gastrointestinal tumours and non-Hodgkin's lymphoma
Bazex's disease	Erythema and hyperkeratosis with scales and itch, predominantly on palms and soles	Head and neck, lung and gastrointestinal tract Men only
Erythroderma		
Erythroderma gyratum repens	Rapidly changing and advancing gyri with scaling and pruritus	Almost always associated with malignancy (often breast or lung)
Flushing	Usually head and neck	Carcinoid, medullary carcinoma of thyroid
Bullous		
Pemphigoid	Large tense bullae with absent acantholysis	Uncertain association with malignancy
Dermatitis Herpetiformis	Sub-epidermal bullae with scarring	Associated with coeliac disease Associated with T cell lymphoma and enteropathy
Miscellaneous		
Dermatomyositis	Purple–pink erythema, especially around eyes	7–50% associated with cancer
Hypertrichosis languginosa	Rapid development of fine downy hair	High association with cancer
Acquired ichthyosis	Generalized dry cracking skin	

Table 19.3 Cutaneous manifestations of malignancy

Non-paraneoplastic causes must be excluded. Anorexia and nausea may be due to treatment or bowel obstruction.

Fever

Pyrexia of unknown origin may be a presenting feature of malignancy. It is usually associated with lymphoma, hypernephroma, osteogenic sarcoma and myxoma. In lymphoma, the presence of fever is an adverse prognostic factor. The cause is probably the release of cytokines and/or pyrogens from the tumour.

Hypertrophic pulmonary osteoarthropathy

This condition is usually associated with adenocarcinoma of the lung, although any primary or metastatic tumour in the chest can be associated with it. However, it is almost non-existent in small cell lung cancer. Patients develop clubbing, periostitis of the long bones and sometimes develop polyarthritis. Periostitis/arthritis tends to involve the distal ends of the tibia, fibula, humerus, radius and ulna.

Amyloid

Amyloid is classically associated with plasma cell malignancies, but it is also associated with Hodgkin's disease, non-Hodgkin's lymphoma, hypernephroma and carcinoma of the cervix and bladder. Amyloid derived from immunoglobulin light chains (AL type) is associated with myeloma. The protein found in chronic disease/malignancy (AA type) is unrelated to any immunoglobulin.

20

Communicating with patients and relatives

A FAULKNER

The diagnosis of cancer is a frightening prospect for most people. The word itself provokes fear and many people associate it with death. Even those who come to grips with the reality of cancer know that they are facing an uncertain future. The role of the health care professional is to help the individual to be as hopeful as possible within realistic boundaries of the disease and the potential for treatment.

Identifying problems

A large body of knowledge has identified the common problems of cancer patients. For example, we know that over 25% of patients following mastectomy will suffer from either body image problems, marital problems and/or clinical anxiety and/or depression. Similarly with stoma patients problems are commonly linked to the change in body image and the fear that the individual will no longer be acceptable to those that they love.

This information can be very useful in alerting health professionals to some of the problems that patients have. However, such information may also blind the workers to other problems that are unique to the individual. Therefore in ascertaining what the patients' problems are, it is important to make no assumptions about particular problems, but to let the individual identify what particularly is worrying him or her.

Many patients, when they are managing to cope with their diagnosis, will describe how they were not given enough information. Clinicians, quite rightly, may feel that they have given a great deal of information to the patient. One of the pitfalls here is that if information is to be absorbed by the patient, it has to be relevant to the patient's needs and pace. Information is often given immediately after the patient has been given the diagnosis. The reason that information is not absorbed at this time is because the patient is very likely to be suffering from shock and may later describe feelings of numbness and unreality.

Communication skills

To help identify patients' problems and to look for a way forward, a skilled approach is required. The patient must be given space to say what he or she needs to say. Only by assessing the individual's needs can the professional communicate effectively with patients and their relatives.

Questioning style

Too often, questions are asked in a closed manner. This means that the patient has only three choices of answer: Yes, No or I don't know. This closed approach is perfectly reasonable if facts are required. In any assessment of a patient there will be a place for closed questions to collect demographic data and check necessary facts. However, when ascertaining what is worrying the patient about the diagnosis and the possible treatment options, a more open approach is required. Open questions are appropriate here to give a wide choice of how to answer. These questions usually start with words such as how, why, tell me, and leave the control with the patient. When assessing a patient, the first question should be open and very broad so that the patient can relate his story in his own way from his own perspective. Later, as the patient talks about his illness, the health professional can make the questions more focused while still leaving them open.

Doctor: Tell me how things have been for you, Mr Smith.

Mr Smith: Well, it was all right until I started this bleeding from my back passage.

Doctor: Tell me about the bleeding.

In the above exchange it will be seen that the first question was very broad and open but the second one focused on the area that the patient had identified.

Encouraging the patient to identify the problems and lead the interaction is called 'following a patient-led agenda'. Such an agenda, however, does not mean that the professional cannot include professional items that have to be covered. For example, if a patient gives an indication that he is depressed, then the doctor would screen for other signs to check if clinical depression is present.

By working in this way a series of problems should be identified which cover most areas of information that the health professional needs to explore. If there are glaring omissions in the patient's story, then the health professional should end the assessment by explaining that there are one or two items that must also be addressed, in order to gain a complete picture of the present situation.

Cues

In following a patient-led agenda, the health professional is presented with cues. For example, Mr Smith gave as his first priority his worry about his bleeding. This cue was picked up by the doctor. Unfortunately all cues are not quite so obvious and the health professional needs to develop the ability to listen to the patient so that cues which are given can be picked up and explored.

Cues are not given in a neat schedule one at a time. Very often the patient will give a number of cues at the same time, covering psychological, social and physical factors. The common behaviour of health professionals is to pick up those cues which are simple to address. For example, Mr Smith may have said things were all right until the end of the holiday and then there was bleeding. The doctor may still have picked up the cue about bleeding, but would be at risk of missing the cue 'end of holiday'.

Missing such cues is often seen in the literature to be bad practice, but in reality, missing cues is not terribly important as long as they are eventually picked up. If a matter is important to a patient he will give the cue more than once. With Mr Smith the doctor may have picked up the cue about bleeding and said, 'Well I can see why that's worrying you so much' and Mr Smith might have responded, 'Well it came on top of what happened at the end of the holiday'. Mr Smith is then giving the doctor a second chance to pick up on what the problem was at the end of the holiday. If the doctor continues to ignore the cue, then the patient may stop mentioning it and a valuable piece of information may be lost.

Sometimes an individual gives so many cues that it is worthwhile for the health professional to make a comment. The doctor might say for example, 'You've given me a lot of information there; you're worried about the bleeding, you're worried about the problem with your wife, you seem to have some financial difficulties. I wonder which of those you'd like to talk about first?' By giving the individual a choice in this way, it can be possible to allow the patient to prioritize what is worrying him most.

This is where assumptions may get in the way; it is possible for the professional carer to believe that cancer is the most important problem for the patient. In reality, it may be something quite different that is of utmost importance for the patient to disclose that will then put feelings about the cancer into a true perspective.

Meaning

It is important, when communicating with cancer patients, to check that there is a clear understanding over meaning, both in terms of the meaning of what is said to the patient and what the patient says to the health professional. There are many ambiguous words in our vocabulary so jargon from health workers must be avoided and jargon used by patients should be checked. For example, the patient who says he is depressed may mean that he is 'fed up' and his meaning could be anything from being simply 'fed up' because he is off work and having to have tests, through to clinical depression where the knowledge of his cancer is giving him suicidal thoughts.

Given these problems, if a patient uses a word that has multiple meanings it is worth asking, 'Can you tell me what you mean by that?' Similarly if the health professional has to use a difficult word, it is not insulting to ask the patient, 'Do you want me to tell you a bit more about what I mean?'. Most patients would welcome such help in a difficult time when they are trying to understand a life-threatening illness and an uncertain future.

Similarly, patients are often quite vague when telling their story, particularly about time scales. Saying that the bleeding happened at the end of a holiday does not tell the health professional when exactly the bleeding started and so it is important to encourage the patient to be precise. If the patient says the bleeding started at the end of his holiday say 'Do you remember exactly when that was?'. Such questions encourage the patient to give exact details and help him to believe that the health professional is interested in every aspect of his disease, and its effect on his life.

Making sense

Non-verbal messages are often as important, if not more so, than what is actually being said. Therefore, inherent in an assessment interview is the matching or mismatching of verbal and non-verbal messages. This 'putting together' of the whole message can often lead to a feeling about what is going on. If this happens and there is a strong feeling, based on the composite message, then action should be taken in terms of testing feelings or hypotheses with the patient. This is called 'making an educated guess' and should only be used if it is based on a strong feeling coming from what is being said by the patient. The patient, for example, may have been describing the time of illness and the impact on family life and by the way he is looking he may give the counsellor a clear feeling that the time has been very difficult. The counsellor might say, 'Mr Smith, I'm getting the impression that you found this all extremely difficult'.

If the professional is correct, the patient will often give a sigh of relief because it is so wonderful to have somebody who understands. If the health professional has not picked up the right messages, then the patient will very often correct and say something like, 'It's not that I found it difficult, I've just been so scared'. In either event the patient will be encouraged to go on talking because he will feel that the health professional is really trying to understand how he is feeling.

Prompting

Not all patients find it easy to talk, even when they are with a skilled counsellor. They may need help to talk and this can best be done by gentle prompting on the part of the health professional along with acknowledgement of the fact that the patient is finding it difficult to talk. For example, if a question is asked which is followed by a silence, it is worth saying something like, 'You seem to find this quite difficult to talk about'. This gives the patient the opportunity to say why it is difficult, or it may give them the chance to say, 'I don't want to talk about this at the moment'. If the patient finds the situation too painful to talk about, then it is often best to leave things and return to the subject at a later date.

Towards the end of the interview, the health professional should summarize and check with the patient that they have indeed identified the problems as they appear to the patient. After this, it is always useful to ask a screening question. It might be 'Well Mr Smith, I think I've got a clear idea of how things are for you. It's unfortunate that your illness has come at a time when you've also got family and financial problems. I wonder given the problems we've identified, is there anything else at all that you want to talk to me about?' This gives the patient the opportunity to disclose worrying problems that simply have not come up during the time of the interview, but which are relevant to the current situation.

Attitudes

Communication skills will only be effective if the health professional has a good positive attitude; towards the patient, the illness and the treatment. This means taking a non-judgemental approach and trying to avoid giving advice or inappropriate reassurance. Early research in this area suggests that most nurses and doctors want to be over-reassuring to their patients and to give them unrealistic hopes for the future. Most patients who have been treated in this way become very bitter, feeling that they have not been trusted with the reality and also that somehow the clinical carer is talking down to them rather than treating them as someone who is tough enough to take bad news.

Bad news

There has been an 'either/or' belief in the past, with some believing that bad news should be broken and others believing it should not. The debate raged for many years. Those who believed in breaking bad news took the view that honesty was the only way forward. Those who felt that bad news should not be broken to a patient felt that hope had to be maintained.

In fact, breaking bad news should be accomplished at the patient's pace if it is to be absorbed. Table 20.1 shows the stages of breaking bad news at a patient's pace. Using this model of warning first, and then pacing the information, makes it possible to stop giving information at any point when the patient identifies that he has had enough. This means that some patients with advanced cancer may die without knowing exactly what is wrong with them. This is their choice. Others may take several attempts before they can finally say, 'Tell me what it is doctor'. Yet others will want to know everything straight away.

Part of the communication skills needed by all health professionals is the ability to identify how much information each individual requires and the period of time

Strategy	Example
Warning shot	Dr: I have had the results of your tests and I'm afraid they are more serious than I hoped.
Pacing	Patient: Serious? Dr: Yes, you have some abnormal cells. Patient: Abnormal – what do you mean? Dr: I'm afraid it's a tumour.
Give space	Dr: Seems as if this is quite a shock to you.
Pick up pieces	Dr: I can see you are upset. Would it help to tell me how you are feeling?

Table 20.1   Breaking bad news

they need to absorb it. It is also important to identify those individuals who cope using denial. This can be a very strong coping mechanism and should not be lightly taken away. The level of denial should be assessed and the health professional should be alert to when the individual is ready to move on.

Hope

Hope is often interpreted to mean 'hope that the patient will recover from their cancer and that the treatment will work'. This rather narrow view can get in the way of working with patients who have advanced cancer and a shortened life expectancy.

A better description of hope is one in which the patient can make the most of the time that they have left. This means setting short-term goals that probably can be reached and, by doing this, the patient's morale is lifted. In setting short-term goals they are motivating themselves to be interested in what is going on around them for the foreseeable future.

Often a patient will set some goal, such as reaching their silver wedding anniversary, seeing their first grandchild born, or something similar, that doctors and other health professionals feel will not be reached. Surprisingly, most patients seem to be very realistic on these occasions and often reach their goals even if they die a day or two later. It is as if, by being motivated to achieve a certain ambition, they will survive and fulfil this particular goal, although there is no scientific evidence for this. The professional carer's attitude should encourage the patient to meet short-term goals that are reasonably realistic.

A difficulty arises when a patient is unrealistic about the future and may set goals that certainly will not be reached. While maintaining a positive attitude, the adviser may be able to help the individual to modify the goals so that they still have something to work for but in a more limited way. In working with hope in this way, there is less likelihood of the patient dying with unfinished business and its aftermath. It is hoped, they will have become realistic enough to talk to relatives and loved ones about what they think will happen and what they want to happen in terms of relationships and in terms of special possessions.

Spiritual issues

If professional health workers communicate effectively with their patients and help the patients to identify their problems, the patient will often be very prepared to disclose quite deep inner feelings to the health professional. In talking about feelings the patient is verbalizing problems, often of a very personal nature. These often include spiritual issues.

Many health professionals are anxious about encouraging patients to disclose their deep feelings. They are worried that they are in fact spying on the most personal part of the patient and somehow intruding into his or her private world. If communication skills are used appropriately and the patient is left in control of how much is disclosed, then it should be possible to accept that what the patient discloses is what he or she chooses to disclose.

Often the feelings are simply verbal disclosure of concerns and do not necessarily have any solution. This is particularly true in spiritual issues. The patient may ask, 'Is there something after this?' 'Is there an afterlife?' or 'How could God treat me like this?' These questions are usually rhetorical and the health professional, by encouraging the patient to talk, will also encourage that patient to make sense, as far as they can, of what is going on.

The role of the health professional when a patient is disclosing feelings is to get a clear picture of what the patient is saying and then lift them back to a less intense feeling and move on to another area. This is commonly called 'lifting' or 'rescuing', but what it means is that rather than allow the patient to wallow in feelings, he or she is encouraged to disclose and discuss them, but then move on to other issues.

Many clinicians are concerned if patients show emotion, as they undoubtedly will, if they are discussing their deeper fears and worries. That the patient will cry is less important than that the health professional will allow the patient to do so and yet move on. Handing a tissue and acknowledging the pain of the fears and worries can help the patient. This is particularly true of the patient who has had no-one to talk to before and really has a need to express her feelings. Such patients will often say after an interview, 'Well I had a good cry but I felt so much better for getting it off my chest'.

Unwinding

It can be seen from this brief chapter that effective communication with patients who are suffering from cancer at any stage can be quite painful. By interacting effectively the health professional will be closer to the patient's pain and it can be concluded that if the patient feels better for getting things off his or her chest the carer may feel temporarily worse because they have taken the patient's burden for themselves. For this reason, carers have to set their own limits on how much emotion they can take from others in any one period of time. This is not a competitive matter, it is personal for each health professional.

One way is to balance the communication elements of the work with other less taxing activities. For example, to go from one patient who has disclosed their fears and worries and their distress straight to another patient will mean that the carer is unlikely to be able to help the second patient as they did the first because they will not have recovered from the reverberations from the first patient. However, if the health professional goes from heavy interaction with a distressed patient to other aspects of the work, they can then go to the second patient who needs to talk in a fresher state of mind.

Many health professionals are helped to deal with the costs of caring for very ill patients by having someone that they can talk to or indeed a support group where problems can be discharged in a safe environment. Unfortunately, hospitals do not always have built-in support mechanisms. In that case, the health professional needs to find someone with whom they can talk who may be able to help them with their worries.

Another help is to balance work and play, so that the workload is left behind at the end of the day; family and friends can help here. Those activities that help an individual to unwind at the end of a working day are usually very personal and can include sport, exercise, relaxation, music and a host of other activities. By switching off in this way, the carer is not being selfish but is ensuring that he or she will be fresh enough to meet the patient's needs the following day and for the period of time that the patient needs them.

21

Palliative and continuing care

J M O'NEILL

In a specialist oncology centre about one-third of patients will be cured. Therefore much of the work of the centre is concerned with the care of patients in the palliative phase of their advanced disease (Table 21.1) when cure is impossible. The period of *palliative and continuing care* incorporates the time from diagnosis of incurable malignancy (or uncontrolled or recurrent disease) to death; life expectancy may be days, months or even years.

The palliative approach to treatment does not rule out active anti-cancer therapy, but patient selection must carefully balance efficacy with potential toxicity. Palliative treatment should give maximum symptomatic relief by the simplest method available with the minimum upset to the patient and in the shortest possible time. There is a change in emphasis from 'cure' to 'care'; from survival to quality of life; and from disease control to symptom control.

The radiotherapist, oncologist and surgical oncologist should form part of a multidisciplinary team including (among others), specialists in palliative medicine, anaesthetists in pain clinics, physiotherapists, nurses and GPs.

In deciding which type of treatment approach might be most helpful to the patient, it is useful to decide which phase of disease he or she is in (Table 21.1). This will indicate which therapies are most relevant to the cancer patient (Table 21.2).

Aims of palliative care

The aim of palliative care is to maximize the quality of the patient's remaining life.

The specialty of palliative medicine focuses on the physical aspects of symptom relief in the overall context of the physical, psychological and social environment of the patient and his or her family. This is a combined team approach in association

Phase	Priority	Treatment toxicity
Curative	Survival	May be high
Palliative	Quality of life	Ideally low
Terminal	Quality of life	Ideally none

Table 21.1 Phases of illness

Disease modifying management
Chemotherapy
Radiotherapy
Surgery

Symptomatic management
Analgesics and adjuvant medications
Anaesthetic and neurosurgical procedures
Non-drug treatments (e.g. TENS, acupuncture)

Comprehensive palliative care service
Hospital, home, hospice

Intensive team approach
Rehabilitation – physiotherapy and occupational therapy, extensive psycho-social support
and bereavement service

Table 21.2   Palliative measures

with other medical and paramedical specialties, such as nursing, social work and
physiotherapy.

Total suffering

The concept of 'total suffering' is important (Figure 21.1). Untreated or unresolved
problems relating to any one cause of suffering may cause or exacerbate other
causes of suffering. Hence the team approach to care is invaluable.

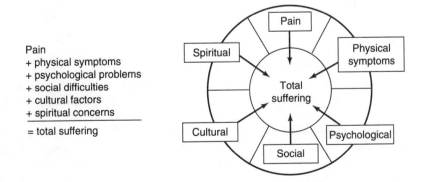

Pain
+ physical symptoms
+ psychological problems
+ social difficulties
+ cultural factors
+ spiritual concerns

= total suffering

Figure 21.1   Total suffering.

1	Hospice in-patient care
	Independent hospices
	Hospital continuing care units (NHS)
	National charities – Macmillan
	Marie Curie
	Sue Ryder
2	Home care services
	Macmillan nursing service
	Marie Curie home care service
3	Hospital teams
	Over 200 hospital teams in UK with support nurses or teams
4	Day hospices
	Over 200 day units now exist
	Allow patients to manage at home whilst maintaining contact with hospice facilities
5	Hospices offering specialist care
	AIDS/HIV – six centres
	Children's hospices – 11 established, ten planned

Table 21.3 Palliative care provision

Good palliative care therefore involves:

- symptom control
- rehabilitation – physiotherapy and occupational therapy
- psychological support
- good communication among the palliative care team
- choice of venue of care (e.g. home, hospice or hospital)
- bereavement support as appropriate.

Services available

Hospice

In January 1995, the Hospice Information Service revealed that there are over 200 in-patient hospice units providing more than 3000 beds for the palliative care of patients in the UK and Ireland. The Palliative Care movement provides care in many settings (Table 21.3).

Hospices admit patients for short-term care for three reasons: symptom control; rehabilitation and respite care (often to give caring relatives a break); or for terminal care. Specialized palliative care units should be likened to *intensive care units* for patients with incurable cancer, for those whose physical symptoms or emotional problems require a high degree of professional input. It is estimated that 40–50 hospice beds are required per million people in the population.

Hospices can also call on a vast army of volunteer and support workers, who assist and support their patients. Hospices have a high staff-to-patient ratio. They act as palliative care training and research centres, are active in the use of complementary treatments and have well-established bereavement support networks.

Home care and day care

It is estimated that a patient with advanced cancer will spend 90% of his or her time under the care of the GP at home. About one-third of patients die in the community.

Home care teams (commonly Macmillan nurses) and Day Hospice Units, both generally based in a hospice, allow patients to spend as much as possible of the last phase of their illness at home, which is where many prefer to die.

Hospital

Of nearly 135 000 patients dying of malignant disease almost 60% die in acute general hospitals. Recent findings in Sheffield demonstrated that, of all cancer deaths in hospital, approximately one-third occurred under the care of each of physicians, surgeons and oncologists.

Hospital support teams

With 60% of patients with far advanced cancer being cared for in acute hospitals, it was a natural extension of the hospice movement to introduce the hospice approach to acute hospitals. This was done through the establishment of hospital support teams.

The team works in an advisory capacity within the hospital providing specialist advice on symptom control and pain relief. The team also gives emotional support to patients and carers with difficult physical and psycho-social problems, as well as playing an important role in education and research within the hospital. The team also liaises with community palliative care services. Most teams comprise two or more Macmillan nurses and many teams are multidisciplinary, including a doctor, social worker and chaplain and have close links with community Macmillan teams and hospices. The first hospital support team was established at St Thomas's Hospital, London, in 1977. In 1995, over 200 hospitals in the UK have support teams or support nurses.

Palliative medicine has been recognized as a separate specialty since 1987, with specific training requirements. This will improve the provision of high standards nationally and should encourage research into palliative care.

Symptom control

The symptoms which most commonly cause problems in management are pain, vomiting, constipation and breathlessness. Patients with progressive, far advanced cancer may have multiple problems, a limited time left in which to be assessed and frequently changing symptoms. As in any other branch of medicine, careful history and examination are important. However, the management of a frail, symptomatic patient may necessitate minimal investigation, the consideration (but rejection) of aggressive therapeutic manoeuvres, such as parenteral nutrition, intravenous antibiotics, major surgery, radiotherapy or chemotherapy, and maximal and prompt treatment.

Pain

Pain is the most common symptom experienced by patients with cancer. Pain is a presenting feature in 30–45% of patients with cancer and occurs in 70% of those with advanced disease. In two-thirds of patients, this pain is caused by the cancer itself. The types of treatment for cancer pain are summarized in Figure 21.2.

Assessment

Pain has both physical and psychological components. Multiple sites of pain are common, with 80% of patients having more than one site of pain. A full physical and psychological history, physical examination and diagnosis of each pain is mandatory.

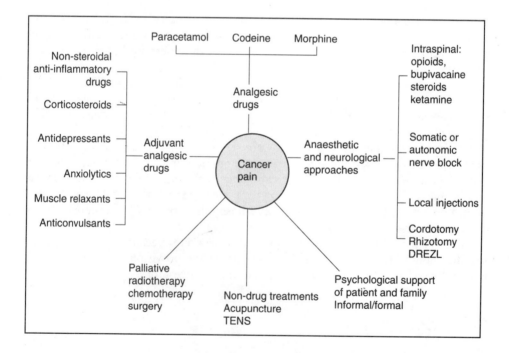

Figure 21.2   Treatment of cancer pain.

Step one	Non-opioids: paracetamol aspirin
Step two	Mild opioids: coproxamol (dextropopoxyphene) codeine dihydrocodeine
Step three	Strong opioids: morphine diamorphine

Table 21.4 WHO pain ladder

Principles of pain treatment

1   Explain treatment to patient and set realistic goals (e.g. pain-free nights initially).
2   Use the World Health Organization (WHO) pain ladder (Table 21.4). Drugs should be given: by mouth (possible in the majority of cases); by the clock (regularly); and by the ladder, as above.

Add adjuvant drugs as necessary. Non-steroidal anti-inflammatory drugs (NSAIDs) should be given for bone pain. Steroids can be given for nerve compression, hepatomegaly and raised intracranial pressure. Tricyclics and anti-convulsants are used for nerve pain.

3   Give analgesic regularly and as often as required for 'breakthrough' pain.
4   Most patients (80–90%) with advanced cancer, attending cancer centres, have their pain controlled with drugs given orally.
5   Adjust the dose upwards until the patient is pain free with minimal side-effects.
6   Address psychological issues if this will raise the pain threshold.
7   Non-drug treatments may be useful, for example radiotherapy for bone meta-stases, nerve blocks for poorly controlled pain and physiotherapy.
8   Regularly review the situation. Doses may need daily alteration initially.

Prescribing morphine

1   Explain the treatment and deal with the patient's anxieties about tolerance and addiction.
2   Discuss common side-effects with the patient. The only persistent side-effect is constipation which occurs in 99% of patients. Prescribe laxatives prophy-lactically to counteract constipation. Drowsiness occurs in 20% of patients, but wears off after a few days. Nausea occurs in 28% of patients, but wears off after a few days. Prescribe anti-emetics if they are needed for 1 week. Dry mouth occurs in 40% of patients. Confusion, which is usually mild and self limiting, occurs in 5% of patients.

Pain syndrome	Type of block
Brachial plexus pain	brachial plexus
Lumbosacral plexus injury	intraspinal
Difficult perineal and pelvic pains	
Painful hip or knee	lumbar psoas
Chest wall pain	intercostal
Upper abdominal pain from gastric or	
Pancreatic cancer (80% response)	coeliac plexus

Table 21.5 Common nerve blocks

3 Increase the dose by at least 30–50% as needed.
4 A double dose may be given at bedtime and the 4 a.m. dose stopped.
5 Morphine, in the form of slow release tablets (MST Continus) is useful when the pain has been controlled and the patient is taking a constant dose of morphine.

Non-oral routes of administration for opioids

Opioids can be given sub-lingually. A strong opioid given by this route is buprenorphine (Temgesic).

Oxycodone suppositories can be given rectally every 8 hours.

Subcutaneous infusion is very useful and commonly used. It avoids the pain of repeated injections. Other drugs can be given in the syringe driver (e.g. some anti-emetics and sedatives). A pharmacist's advice may be necessary.

Intraspinal diamorphine can be very useful for patients whose pain is responsive to opioids but who are troubled by systemic side-effects, especially sedation caused by the high doses they require.

Other treatment modalities

Palliative radiotherapy is useful for bone metastases and is often given as a single fraction. Pain relief response is achieved in 50% of patients at 2 weeks and 80% at 4 weeks.

Transcutaneous electrical nerve stimulation and acupuncture are often effective, but pain relief may be short lived.

Nerve blocks (usually with a local anaesthetic) are indicated for localized pain where high doses of opioids are ineffective. Common clinical indications are shown in Table 21.5.

Nausea and vomiting

In far advanced cancer, 42% of patients suffer nausea and 32% vomiting. Patients find nausea almost as distressing as pain. Nausea and vomiting may originate from cancer within the gastrointestinal tract, or from stimulation of the CNS.

CNS causes

The vomiting centres (emetic centres) in the medulla are the final common pathway for many cases of nausea and vomiting. They are rich in histamine and muscarinic cholinergic receptors and therefore cyclizine is useful for treating nausea arising from many causes. Vagal afferents from visceral structures feed into these centres and the anticholinergic drug hyoscine hydrobromide is a useful second-line agent, though it can be very sedating.

If nausea due to intracranial pressure fails to respond to dexamethasone, cyclizine is a useful adjuvant. Nausea related to motion should also respond to cyclizine.

The chemoreceptor trigger zone lying in the floor of the fourth ventricle, close to the emetic centre, contains chemoreceptors which sample blood and CSF. It is therefore responsible for nausea and vomiting due to blood-borne causes, such as drugs (particularly opioids), biochemical abnormalities (e.g. hypercalcaemia and uraemia), toxins, and nausea due to disseminated cancer.

There is a high concentration of dopamine receptors in this area, hence the logic for choosing a potent dopamine antagonist, such as haloperidol. It has a long action (half-life of 16 hours) so that a once daily dose is sufficient in most patients. Prochlorperazine is an alternative, but has an unpredictable oral absorption rate.

Gastric causes

The most commonly neglected cause of nausea and vomiting is untreated constipation. Delayed intestinal emptying may respond to gastric-motility agents such as metoclopramide, domperidone or cisapride.

Gastric irritation may be caused by drugs (e.g. NSAIDs, antibiotics and iron) and these should be stopped if necessary; antacids and H_2-blocking drugs may be helpful. The nausea of intestinal obstruction may be reduced by haloperidol, cyclizine, metoclopramide and methotrimeprazine (a phenothiazine with marked sedative properties).

Constipation

Constipation is very common in patients with advanced cancer, it should always be looked for. A supine X-ray can be invaluable in cases which are difficult to assess. It is caused mainly by poor oral intake, immobility and drug therapy. Opioids and drugs which reduce bowel contraction by their anticholinergic action (e.g. antidepressants, cyclizine and phenothiazine) are the main drugs causing constipation.

Prevention is better than cure. All patients commencing opioids should have regular daily laxatives and the dose should be tailored to give a comfortable bowel motion every 2–3 days. A popular drug is co-danthrusate in capsule form, which is a combination of stool softener and stimulant.

A '3-day-rule' should apply for rectal measures. If the patient has not had a bowel movement for 3 days, despite regular oral laxatives, rectal measures should be instituted. Glycerine and bisacodyl suppository should be given initially.

Control of respiratory symptoms

Dyspnoea is a common, frightening and undertreated symptom in patients with advanced cancer. Reversible causes of dyspnoea should be treated as long as worthwhile benefit results. Unless the patient's poor general condition precludes it: cardiac failure should be treated with diuretics; anaemia treated with transfusions; chest infections with antibiotics and physiotherapy; and bronchospasm with bronchodilators, preferably nebulized. Pleural effusions should be tapped and steroids (e.g. dexamethasone) used for radiation pneumonitis and carcinomatous lymphangitis.

Radiotherapy should be considered in all cases, and though there may be no radiographic impression of change in tumour mass after treatment, ventilation/perfusion 'mismatch' may be improved, and compression of pulmonary blood and lymphatic vessels may be relieved.

The mainstay of symptomatic management is low-dose opioid therapy (e.g. morphine liquid), which acts centrally to reduce the sensation of dyspnoea and has been shown to improve the overall activity level of many patients. Where the patient is on morphine for pain, the dose should be increased by 50% to relieve dyspnoea. Respiratory depression is minimal, provided doses are adjusted slowly, maintaining a respiratory rate greater than 10 per minute. The morphine also suppresses cough, the other distressing symptom that patients with lung involvement often complain of.

Small doses of benzodiazepine (e.g. diazepam) may be helpful when anxiety is a major feature. Oxygen by nasal prongs may be helpful if the patient is hypoxic.

Simple measures, such as a reasonably cool and spacious room, with a free flow of air, assisted by a fan, and appropriate explanation and reassurance to patient and family, are essential aspects of management.

The terminal phase

As death approaches, the focus of care changes. Relatives and staff need time for changes in prognosis and management to be explained in a caring and unhurried fashion.

Intravenous infusions should be stopped when appropriate, as they may unnecessarily prolong the dying process. Bronchial secretions (death rattle) can be dried by giving hyoscine hydrobromide subcutaneously, mainly for the relatives' comfort as the patient is often deeply unconscious. General discomfort and stiffness in immobile patients can be relieved by a pressure mattress and NSAID suppositories. Unnecessary medications should be stopped and essential analgesics and other drugs given by the most comfortable route.

Terminal restlessness may be due to unrelieved pain, hypoxia, a distended bladder or rectum, but frequently no cause can be identified. The following drugs can be combined in a continuous subcutaneous infusion: diamorphine for pain; hyoscine for 'death rattle'; midazolam or methotrimeprazine for agitation; diazepam suppositories are also useful.

Relatives will need regular reassurance and explanation throughout the final illness, and selective follow-up by the hospital bereavement service, often co-ordinated by the social work department.

The deceased patient's GP should be informed of the death by the next working day.

A brief review with other staff members of the success (or otherwise) of the management of the final phase of the patient's illness will help to maintain high standards of care of the terminally ill patient.

22

Oncological emergencies

B W HANCOCK

Superior vena cava obstruction

The syndrome of superior vena cava obstruction usually results from pressure on the superior vena cava by tumour masses in the superior mediastinum. Occasionally, it is due to actual tumour involvement of the vessel and mural thrombus formation. The most common cause is lymph node metastases from a primary carcinoma of the bronchus. It is much less common from node enlargement by lymphoma, or from thymoma or other mediastinal tumours. Development of the syndrome may be gradual or rapid; in the latter case, superimposed thrombosis is the likely cause.

Classically, there is over-filling and distension of the veins of the head, neck and upper limbs, and dilated subcutaneous veins over the front of the chest and of the abdomen, the latter being a manifestation of collateral circulation to the inferior vena cava. There is associated oedema of tissues, and in severe cases suffusion of the conjunctivae.

Initial responses to radiation or chemotherapy are often good. It is an observed fact that only partial regression of the mediastinal mass can lead to complete regression of the signs of obstruction. Thrombosis of the superior vena cava will not respond to irradiation, also it seldom responds to conventional anti-coagulant therapy; stenting may be beneficial (Chapter 3). When radiotherapy is the method of choice this should be fractionated; in severe cases, the dose for the first exposure may be increased with the aim of gaining a more rapid response. Development of superior vena cava obstruction from bronchial carcinoma carries a bad prognosis, the average survival being 4–6 months.

Progressive obstruction to the main bronchi or lower trachea with stridor also presents as an emergency situation. Rapid symptomatic improvement usually follows radiation therapy, especially for small cell carcinoma of the bronchus. For sensitive tumours, cytotoxic chemotherapy may be equally effective. In the acute phase, dexamethasone may also be helpful.

Spinal cord compression

Evidence of spinal cord compression may indicate a surgical emergency. Pressure from tumour masses within the spinal canal, or from vertebral body collapse from metastatic involvement, will lead to local ischaemia and to degeneration of nerve fibres if this is severe or prolonged. Degeneration of non-myelinated fibres within the cord is permanent and recovery does not occur. Partial ischaemia, however, is compatible with some degree of recovery of function if the pressure is relieved. Therefore, decompression is indicated as quickly as possible.

If the lesion is a primary one, surgical decompressive laminectomy must be considered, especially if this can be undertaken within 48 hours of development of the condition.

Secondary tumour deposits present a less well-defined situation. If the prognosis for the primary tumour is not bad, and the deposit appears to be solitary, laminectomy is to be recommended. On the other hand, the presence of multiple bony lesions in the spine or of extensive bone destruction locally, may argue against surgical intervention. In such cases, dexamethasone therapy may be of value in limiting reactive oedema. Local palliative radiation therapy will usually reduce associated pain and may produce sufficient tumour regression to allow some recovery of function. The use of high-energy radiation has the advantage of producing less skin reaction, and this may be of great benefit for patients requiring prolonged nursing in bed.

Cytotoxic chemotherapy may be of limited value, but only for very sensitive tumours, such as small cell carcinoma of the bronchus, or lymphoma if this is extradural, or in situations where there is not immediate access to surgery or radiation therapy.

Altered consciousness

As in any branch of medicine, coma of apparently unknown cause is a not uncommon problem in oncology. It is important not to jump to the immediate conclusion that altered consciousness (varying from drowsiness or confusion, to full blown coma) is due to some manifestation of the cancer. The 'pressure' effects of secondary deposits may be responsible, but it is important to exclude other potentially remediable causes.

Status epilepticus resulting from cerebral secondary deposits can lead to profound coma. Good recovery is possible with appropriate anti-convulsant therapy.

Drug overdose (deliberate or iatrogenic) is a particular problem where strong opiate analgesics are being used. A history of escalating doses to combat increasing pain or of anxiety/depression and suicidal thoughts may be obtained; constricted pupils are an additional clue. This situation responds dramatically to intravenous naloxone, an opiate antagonist.

Acute, and less often, chronic (e.g. tuberculous) infection may cause diagnostic difficulties. Toxic confusional states are not uncommon. Pyrexia is usually present to aid diagnosis.

Metabolic disturbance, as a manifestation of the cancer or its treatment, is often reversible. Hyperglycaemia should be looked for when steroids are used. Hypercalcaemia and hyponatraemia, particularly when acute or rapidly progressive, can cause bizarre cerebral features culminating in coma.

Cerebral vascular accidents may occur coincidentally or as a complication of associated haematological abnormalities (e.g. thrombocytopenia).

Hypercalcaemia

Hypercalcaemia may be a feature of many cancers, and as we have seen is not necessarily associated with overt bone involvement. If slow in onset, it may be asymptomatic. More rapidly developing hypercalcaemia presents with gastro-intestinal disturbances (particularly anorexia, nausea, vomiting and constipation), mental confusion (with drowsiness, psychosis or even coma) or renal failure. In the acute management of hypercalcaemia, saline rehydration is of paramount importance together with efforts to treat the underlying cancer. If rehydration alone is not successful, bisphosphonates are now the treatment of choice. These agents inhibit the osteoclast-mediated bone reabsorption associated with neoplastic activation.

Hyponatraemia

Hyponatraemia *per se* is not uncommon (Chapter 16). It only rarely requires urgent correction, though in its more florid forms therapy consists of restriction of fluid intake together with the administration of demeclocycline (a tetracycline believed to act by blocking the renal tubular effect of antidiuretic hormone) or the administration of sodium chloride, either by mouth or by saline infusion. Treatment of the underlying neoplasm, if possible, is of paramount importance.

Infection

As we have seen, patients with cancer, particularly those involving the lymphoreticular and haematological systems may have defects in immunity and these may be exaggerated by the effects of radiotherapy and chemotherapy. Consequently, infections of various sorts are a constant source of worry.

One common problem encountered in oncology is the patient with pyrexia. Rarely, this can be a feature of the tumour itself (e.g. Hodgkin's disease and renal carcinoma). It is seldom the result of tumour necrosis after treatment. Much more often it is a direct consequence of infection, particularly in patients who are myelo-suppressed (and/or neutropenic) as a result of therapy. The infection may be ill-localized and pyrexia the only outward sign, apart from the patient being ill. Any infective agent may cause pyrexia but often a common pathogen is the offender. Septicaemia is an oncological emergency. It has a high mortality rate and is easily missed or the diagnosis delayed. The policy must be to culture whatever specimen is available (perhaps most importantly the blood) and to initiate empirical treatment with broad-spectrum antibiotics. Though Gram-positive organisms (such as *Staphylococcus epidermidis*) have now become the dominant aetiological agent in causing sepsis, especially in the presence of indwelling intravenous catheters, it is the Gram-negative bacteria, especially *Pseudomonas aeruginosa*, that are associated with high mortality. A common first choice of empiric treatment is the combination of an aminoglycoside (such as gentamicin) plus an anti-pseudomonal penicillin (e.g. piperacillin). Treatment is continued for at least 48 hours after the pyrexia has settled. If the patient remains pyrexial a change of antibiotic may be necessary or even the introduction of an antifungal (e.g. amphotericin B) or antiviral (e.g. acyclovir) therapy, depending on the clinical and microbiological findings. Haematopoietic growth factors are not routinely of help in neutropenic sepsis, unless the period of neutropenia is inordinately prolonged; a situation in which persistent and sinister infections may arise. Severe herpes simplex and herpes zoster/varicella infections mandate intravenous acyclovir and cytomegalovirus gancyclovir. With systemic fungal infections, agents such as fluconazole (*Candida*) or amphotericin (*Aspergillus*) must be given parenterally. For *Pneumocystis* high-dose co-trimoxazole is usually effective.

23

The purchase and provision of hospital-based cancer services

B D AIRD and H C ORCHARD

It is the right of each person in the UK who develops cancer to have 'access to a uniformly high quality of care in the community or hospital wherever they may live'. This is the first principle of *A Policy Framework for Commissioning Cancer Services*, a report by the Expert Advisory Group on Cancer (EAGC), published in April 1995 (known as the Calman Report). This chapter takes a brief look at how hospital services in the National Health Service (NHS) measure up to the spirit of this principle. It also discusses how services might be organized in future, to improve the quality of care that is provided to the large number of people in the UK who will develop cancer at some point in their life.

The present network of cancer services

The current pattern of services, and the way in which they are purchased has developed in a relatively *ad hoc* manner and is now recognized by many health care professionals to be inadequate for the provision of modern comprehensive care for patients with cancer. Cancer services do not fit easily into the purchaser/provider framework of the NHS. The complex nature of the disease means that there are a variety of settings in which care can be most appropriately provided at different stages of illness. A patient may receive treatment from a large number of health care professionals working for various different organizations and at different levels of specialization. At the primary level, care is provided by GPs, district nurses and other specialist nurses. Chest physicians, general surgeons, urologists, gynaecologists and haematologists provide the bulk of secondary care from local district general hospitals. Tertiary services are provided by cancer specialists, such as clinical oncologists (radiotherapists) and medical oncologists, in specialist oncology units, which may be part of teaching hospitals, or independent NHS Trusts. In addition, the high profile nature of the disease attracts much support from the voluntary and charitable sectors, who form a significant body of small service providers which, to a greater or lesser degree, are privately funded. The potential involvement of so many agencies in the treatment of one patient can lead to fragmentation in the delivery of care and difficulties in maintaining any sense of continuity. There are also disadvantages for the purchaser as specific aspects of care are bought from separate providers, and the overall view of the requirements of groups of patients with a particular disease type can be lost. The framework by which hospital services are purchased and provided, and some of its inherent problems are discussed below.

Purchasing hospital-based cancer care

The purchasing of cancer care is managed through the same mechanism as most other aspects of clinical service in the NHS – the contracting cycle. The cycle begins with the purchaser determining the health-care priorities of its resident population and publishing its intentions in its Annual Purchasing Plan. Currently, the only purchasers of tertiary cancer care are District Health Authorities (DHAs) as GP fundholders do not receive funding to buy these services. They do, however, purchase care within the secondary setting and, with moves in the foreseeable future towards total purchasing for GP fundholders, it is probable that GPs will gain responsibility for purchasing an increasing range of care for patients with cancer. Nevertheless, it is likely that there will always be some aspects of cancer care (the high cost and low volume treatments) which are purchased on a DHA basis.

DHAs assess their purchasing priorities in conjunction with imperatives that have been determined locally and set nationally. The national imperatives that play a large part in influencing the purchaser's agenda for cancer services are those specified in the government's *Health of the Nation* initiative. Cancers were a major area focused on by this document, with targets being set for reductions in death rates for breast and lung cancer and the incidence of cervical and skin cancers. The very act of attempting to set targets highlighted the problem of the lack of data on the outcomes of cancer treatment and the difficulties in measuring the effects of treatment interventions. Most purchasers have begun to address the relevant targets in their Annual Purchasing Plans. It is generally the case, however, that although the targets specify that reductions in death rates should be made, as well as halting or reducing incidence, thus far purchasers have generally concentrated their efforts on prevention and screening. Priorities for investment have therefore revolved around health-promotion initiatives and screening services rather than on improved treatment options for people who already have cancer.

Local imperatives are determined primarily by the health needs assessment work undertaken by DHA public health clinicians. If a DHA discovers that its incidence of a particular type of cancer is above the national average and consequently chooses to target additional resources into this area, its choice of the provider with whom to place the annual contract will generally have been made on a historical basis. More recently, and largely as a result of GP involvement, purchasers have begun to identify areas in which a shift in the type or location of care for a group of patients is judged to be desirable and to begin the gradual implementation of such policies. One example of this might be a strategy to enable cancer patients in the terminal stages to die at home, if they so wish, rather than in a hospital or hospice, and consequently to purchase an increased level of community nursing services.

Contracts in their present format do not tell a purchaser very much about what they are actually buying, nor do they give much indication of the quality of care. In particular, treatment provided at secondary level is generally swallowed up within the overall medical and surgical contracts held by the hospital. Contracts with tertiary units often provide little more than an indication of the number of patients treated without specifying how they were treated or what they were treated for. Contracting currencies, which may be expressed in Finished Consultant Episodes or bed days, day cases and out-patient attendances, do not reflect the case mix of patients. An increase in the number of patients needing complex treatment requiring a high level of technical support or complex chemotherapy regimens, with the consequent resource implications, is therefore not addressed by the contracting framework for cancer. A serious stumbling block, however, in the development of more effective contracts is the lack of knowledge and understanding on the part of purchasers about oncology treatment. This is partly due to the fact that, until recently, most specialist cancer treatments have been purchased on a regional basis and so DHAs have not had to grapple with the problems inherent in oncology services. It is exacerbated by the speed and range of developments in treatments. Technological advances in radiotherapy and increasingly sophisticated chemotherapy regimens are continually improving the treatment options for cancer patients. In order for purchasers to increase their effectiveness, a programme of continuing education and updating is therefore necessary.

Providing secondary and tertiary cancer care

While it is generally the case that the first health professional the cancer patient comes into contact with is the GP, the majority of his or her treatment will take place in secondary and tertiary settings. A significant amount of treatment is provided within district general hospitals by clinicians who are specialists in their own right, such as gynaecologists, but are unlikely to have had any formal specialist training in the non-surgical management of cancer. The contribution of these clinicians is primarily surgical, with the specialization being 'organ specific'. For example, a surgeon may specialize in bowel surgery and carry out a variety of malignant and non-malignant work, rather than specializing in surgery related to cancer. In addition, a substantial amount of chemotherapy is prescribed in hospitals by doctors who are not cancer specialists, giving rise to some concern about the quality assurance of such treatment. Clinical haematologists also play a large part in the administration of chemotherapy to patients with leukaemia. Recent guidelines by the Royal College of Radiologists and Royal College of Physicians entitled *Quality Assurance in Cancer Chemotherapy* have been issued in order to try to limit the amount of chemotherapy provided in less than ideal circumstances in non-specialist environments.

Tertiary services are provided at oncology centres which, for the most part, offer radiotherapy, medical oncology and sophisticated diagnostic facilities. They may also have specialist surgical services, bone marrow transplantation facilities and facilities for treating paediatric cancers. Clinical and medical oncologists are supported by a range of other specialists in radiation physics and cytotoxic pharmacy. Research and development into improved treatments for cancer are extremely important to tertiary hospitals. A good centre may have 50 clinical trials under way at any one time, involving approximately 500 patients. The majority of trials are centred around various chemotherapy regimens and receive a high level of resourcing from pharmaceutical companies.

At least one tertiary centre exists in each Region. Centralized planning has played a part in the location of most radiotherapy departments owing to the high capital cost of the equipment. Nevertheless, there are anomalies, with some places being served by two centres relatively close together and others serving large geographical areas. This means that there is inequality of access, with some patients having to travel long distances for radiotherapy and chemotherapy treatment on an out-patient basis. Many tertiary centres run out-patient clinics in their local district general hospitals, with the oncologist travelling out to see new patients referred by clinicians from the peripheral hospital and offering follow-up patients the opportunity to be seen locally. The frequency of these outreach arrangements varies between the different centres, with visits ranging from several times per week to once a month. The opportunity for oncologists to increase the level of service provided on a local basis exists and is likely to be explored further in the near future.

The present framework of secondary and tertiary cancer care in the UK contains many areas of excellence, but a major concern to purchasers and providers alike is that these high standards are not replicated throughout the service. The fragmented way in which services have developed over the last few decades has resulted in inequality of access to timely specialist treatment for some sections of the population. Clearly the number of patients affected by this disease and the associated resource implications demanded a revision of existing systems and the development of a new model to manage the delivery of comprehensive care to cancer patients.

The future integrated network of hospital care

As was mentioned at the beginning of this chapter, 1995 saw the publication of a report of the Expert Advisory Group on Cancer, entitled *A Policy Framework for Commissioning Cancer Services*. The purpose of this document was to establish a pattern of purchasing cancer services (and therefore by implication a pattern of service delivery) which ensured that patients with cancer were detected, diagnosed and treated in the most appropriate place and as early as possible.

To achieve this objective, the Report proposed that care should be purchased at three levels:

- primary care
- designated cancer units
- designated cancer centres.

The primary care level was seen as the focus of care; the expectation being that links between GPs and secondary hospital services would be strengthened and appropriate patterns of referral and follow-up would be established.

Designated cancer units in local hospitals were proposed, which would be of sufficient size to support multidisciplinary clinical teams, with sufficient expertise and facilities to manage the more common cancers. Each cancer unit would require a local co-ordinator to ensure that services dovetailed and that appropriate levels of expertise were being applied across the service. The co-ordinator would also be expected to ensure that non-surgical oncology services, mostly provided on a visiting basis, linked in with the local surgical services. The implications of this model include the need for further sub-specialization in surgery (to ensure that any doctor practising cancer surgery undertook a minimum caseload) and the inevitability that not all general hospitals would be capable of becoming cancer units in their own right.

Designated cancer centres were to provide an extra range of specialized services at the tertiary level in support of cancer units. They would also treat less common cancers or provide treatments which were too technically demanding, too specialized or too capital intensive for cancer units. These cancer centres would normally serve a population in excess of one million people and would be characterized by a high degree of specialization and comprehensive provision of all the facets of cancer care necessary in modern cancer management.

The Report also proposed a further subcategory, a cancer unit with radiotherapy, where, primarily for geographical reasons, it would be necessary to provide radiotherapy services in a cancer unit which was not large enough to support the full range of activity of a cancer centre.

One result of these proposals is an inevitable emphasis on the development of the so called 'hub and spoke' model of provision, where the hub is the cancer centre and the spokes are outreach from the centre to the cancer units. In order to achieve the benefits of a high degree of specialization, in addition to local provision, this model demands that the cancer centre provides non-surgical oncology expertise in the cancer unit (a minimum of five sessions per week was the recommendation), as well as outreach chemotherapy services. In the opposite direction, one would expect to see the rarer and more complex cancers being referred quickly from the cancer unit to the cancer centre.

It is clear that simply designating cancer units and cancer centres will not in itself achieve the benefits of local provision and high specialization along with appropriate referral. This can only be made possible through the development of clinical guidelines and protocols that describe the clinical relationships between different levels of care and deal with the way in which particular disease sites should be handled in relation to diagnosis, treatment and continuing care. The development of these guidelines must obviously be led by doctors and include primary, secondary and tertiary levels to ensure that the patient's needs are catered for in a seamless and continuous service.

From the purchasing perspective, once these guidelines are established it is possible to begin to think seriously in terms of purchasing 'packages of care' which span the whole spectrum of care from primary, through secondary to tertiary and back to the community. This is an attractive proposition to purchasers, who are concerned to ensure that the patient has access to a comprehensive and integrated range of services delivered in the appropriate place and at the appropriate time. It also opens up the possibility, in the longer term, of linking purchasing strategies directly to health outcomes.

From the provider perspective, it opens the door to the creation of highly specialized service providers delivering a range of care through contracts and subcontracts in a variety of locations, freed from the constraints of existing physical or Trust boundaries. This notion of a specialist provider delivering services in a 'shop within a shop' is common enough in the private sector but has yet to make an impact on the NHS.

Challenges ahead for purchasers and providers

It is clear that if purchasers and providers are to succeed in implementing the recommendations of the Calman Report, many difficult challenges will need to be tackled over the next few years. Quite apart from the logistics of shifting to this pattern of purchasing and provision, some of the biggest implications are likely to be:

- The need to challenge existing clinical practice, especially surgical practice to achieve the desirable degree of sub-specialization.

- The need for an increased number of oncology specialists to deliver what is essentially a much higher standard of care and treatment. At the present time, medical manpower plans have not allowed for this increase and, given the lead time necessary to create additional doctors, this presents an enormous challenge to the health-care system. The problem of availability of medical staff will be further exacerbated by the mandatory process of reaccreditation for consultants.

- The need to designate or accredit cancer units and cancer centres in a way which avoids a checklist or 'pass/fail' mentality, and supports their development along agreed pathways and to defined timescales.

- The need to develop adequate data collection mechanisms. Information provision for contracting in cancer care is crude and patchy. The development of clinical guidelines and 'packages of care' will only benefit purchasing and provision if it is underpinned by more flexible, more comprehensive and more robust information systems. Purchasers need population data on the expected number of new and prevalent cases. Health services need data to quantify the anticipated activity and workload by specialty and provider. Data will also be required to evaluate interventions, services and outcomes.

- The cost implications, which are likely to be substantial. While much can be achieved by better organization, there are other aspects such as increased consultant staffing, improved multidisciplinary and multi-site audit, and better information which will all be resource intensive.

The challenges will not, however, simply be of an organizational or clinical nat-ure. Decisions of an economic and ethical character will be unavoidable if services are to be radically improved. The rise in public awareness about health in general and new treatments in particular (with the subsequent demand for them to be avail-able on the NHS), coupled with the gradual increase in the incidence of cancer in the population, will force purchasers to examine their priorities for resource consumption. A clear commitment to purchase on the basis of *need* rather than *demand* is required, but this will be politically and ethically sensitive. The concept of rationing is a particularly difficult one to apply to cancer, which is an emergency specialty with a high proportion of palliative, non-curative work. Providers are, however, already expected to identify areas for 'disinvestment' where specific treatments are not of proven effectiveness, in order that purchasers can withdraw funds to re-invest elsewhere in the system. The lack of available data on the outcomes of cancer treatment, as well as the close relationship between research and service provision, with clinical trials (by their very nature 'unproven') playing such an important role, renders this a hazardous undertaking.

The key to achieving success in these areas will lie partly in the availability and use of improved information on the number and type of procedures undertaken and their effectiveness, as determined by clinical audit. However, the volume of work to be undertaken to establish robust protocols that are acceptable to clinicians and usable within a purchasing framework is immense and will require further investment and collaborative working between DHAs and all providing sectors. The challenge for all parties will be in keeping pace with the continual evolution and change in the field of cancer treatment even while 'packages of care' are being specified, in order that meaningful contracting mechanisms can be developed that reflect what actually happens to the patient and the consequent resource implications. This may result in the establishment of purchasing consortia or 'lead purchaser' arrangements for cancer, in order that the vast knowledge necessary for effective purchasing is concentrated in specific areas, and the number of parties with which cancer centres have to contract is reduced.

The programme for change in the organization of services over the next 5 years is enormous. It represents a real opportunity for clinicians and managers to improve the quality and accessibility of services for patients. This opportunity will be missed unless purchasers and providers develop mature relationships enabling them to work alongside each other to implement the necessary changes. A spirit of co-operation will need to replace the one of aggressive competition that currently exists between many Trusts if networks are to be established and expertise shared, so that the greatest benefit can be realized for patients.

Index